Green Smoothies

FOR

DUMMIES®

A Wiley Brand

by Jennifer Thompson

D1318939

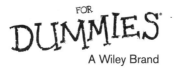

FOR

DUMMIES®

A Wiley Brand

Green Smoothies **For Dummies®**

Published by: **John Wiley & Sons, Inc.,** 111 River Street, Hoboken, NJ 07030-5774, www.wiley.com

Copyright © 2014 by John Wiley & Sons, Inc., Hoboken, New Jersey

Published simultaneously in Canada

For general information on our other products and services, please contact our Customer Care Department within the U.S. at 877-762-2974, outside the U.S. at 317-572-3993, or fax 317-572-4002. For technical support, please visit www.wiley.com/techsupport.

Wiley publishes in a variety of print and electronic formats and by print-on-demand. Some material included with standard print versions of this book may not be included in e-books or in print-on-demand. If this book refers to media such as a CD or DVD that is not included in the version you purchased, you may download this material at http://booksupport.wiley.com. For more information about Wiley products, visit www.wiley.com.

Library of Congress Control Number: 2014935509

ISBN: 978-1-118-87116-4

ISBN 978-1-118-87116-4 (pbk); ISBN 978-1-118-87101-0 (ebk); ISBN 978-1-118-87127-0 (ebk)

Manufactured in the United States of America

10 9 8 7 6 5 4 3 2 1

Contents at a Glance

Table of Contents

Recipes at a Glance

Green Smoothies for Chronic or Serious Medical Conditions 179

Green Smoothies to Maximize Your Workouts ... 205

Introduction

I've been making green smoothies and teaching classes on them for several years now, and I still get excited every time I talk about them because I know they work and I've seen the results. I started making green smoothies after a few years of eating a raw food diet, and I was really impressed with my personal transformation. In just a few days, I felt major improvements in my digestion, energy levels, and overall well-being.

I knew I had to share my success, so I started telling my clients in their health coaching sessions and giving recipe information in my general nutrition and detox lectures. Before I knew it, I was teaching green smoothies classes from my house, and by word-of-mouth, it spread like wildfire. My class became so popular so quickly that I ran out of chairs, and my students had to sit on the floor. At the end of each class, I encouraged them to go out and reclaim their health and the health of the world, one green smoothie at a time.

Looking back, I know it all sounds a bit corny, but guess what? My students went home and started making green smoothies, and their health improved. In fact, the success stories started pouring in, including relief of joint pain, improved eyesight, clearing skin, reversal of digestive problems, increased energy, better sleep, reduced symptoms of menstrual pain and menopause, faster healing from surgery, balanced blood pressure, younger appearance, and even getting pregnant after years of IVF — all just from having a green smoothie every day. It was amazing. Green smoothies exceeded even my expectations of what they could do to improve people's health.

And now I'm excited to have this opportunity to share everything I know about green smoothies with you. By reading this book, you're becoming a green smoothie expert and ambassador. You can explore new ingredients, find out how to prepare the best-tasting green smoothies, personalize your smoothie for your specific health goals, and celebrate the next health success story, in you!

About This Book

Green Smoothies For Dummies is packed with everything you need to know about green smoothies. My goal is give you fast and easy ways to add more fresh leafy greens into your diet with tasty green smoothie recipes. At the same time, I highlight the health benefits of each ingredient so you understand why and how it can improve your health. Knowing what to drink every day and why gives you everything you need to make your daily green smoothie a successful healthy habit for life.

This book includes approximately 100 fast and easy recipes in addition to valuable information to make you an absolute green smoothie expert in no time. And you don't have to read it straight through from beginning to end to get there. Feel free to jump around, dive in to any chapter, and find the stuff that interests you most. I've included cross-references throughout the book to easily direct you back to more a detailed explanation in case you need it. You'll see nutritional information, useful tips, practical advice, and even historical facts put together in an easy-to-read format. And hopefully, this book is kind of fun too. When you discover how to use your food as your medicine, you can get better more quickly and hopefully stay healthy for life.

Although this book is full of valuable and useful information and I encourage you to read it all, you can skip certain sections if you're pressed for time. Each chapter includes helpful and interesting information. You'll see many sidebars in the shaded boxes throughout this book. You may miss an interesting tidbit or fascinating story if you skip them, but you won't miss any must-have knowledge on green smoothies.

In the recipe sections, you'll find variations on some recipes. These are suggestions on how to change a recipe by replacing an ingredient with an alternative option or trying an interesting swap for a different taste. This information isn't crucial, but if you're interested in experimenting with some ingredients, you may want to check out the variations and give them a try.

Foolish Assumptions

I don't make a lot of assumptions about you or your intentions in picking up this book, but if you're here, I'm guessing that one or more of the following statements applies to you:

✔ You've heard the hype and seen some photos of these strangely colored smoothies, and you want to know what they are and how to make them.

✔ You want to make improvements in your diet by adding more natural, whole, or even raw foods, but you don't want to be a full-time gourmet chef.

✔ You're interested in losing weight, gaining energy, looking younger, feeling better, and living longer.

✔ You have a blender and you're ready to give it some lovin'.

✔ You're a busy parent (or parent-to-be) and want fast and easy recipes to keep your family healthy.

✔ You're supporting a friend or family member who's recovering from illness, and you're looking for nutrition tips and healthy recipes to share.

✔ You want to know more about the how, what, and why of detox, superfoods, green smoothies, and raw food.

✔ You've already starting making green smoothies but want new ideas, tips, and recipes to get them tasting great.

Icons Used in This Book

To make this book easier to navigate, I include the following icons to help you find key information about green smoothies:

 You'll see this icon when I want you to pay special attention to an important piece of information. Remember, this icon highlights points to remember!

 The Tip icon is a sign for practical information and ideas to help you save time, make better smoothies, and keep your equipment in tip-top shape.

 The Warning icon marks important health, allergy, or safety information related to equipment and/or ingredients. When you see this icon, you know to take care with the subject at hand.

 I don't use this icon often, but when I do, it highlights some technical trivia or historical facts that you may find interesting.

 This icon points out bonus material you can find online.

Beyond the Book

In addition to the information and recipes in the print or e-book you're reading right now, this product also comes with some access-anywhere goodies on the web. Check out the free Cheat Sheet at www.dummies.com/cheatsheet/greensmoothies for helpful insight on what makes a green smoothie, how green smoothies can help you meet your health goals, and pointers on boosting your smoothies with superfoods.

At www.dummies.com/extras/greensmoothies, you can find more free information about green smoothies, including common mistakes to avoid when blending them up, how to get your whole family excited about your green smoothie revolution, and a one-week snapshot of groceries and easy menus to get you started. You can also discover the top ten reasons you should be drinking green smoothies, in case you're still on the fence.

Where to Go from Here

One of the best features of the *For Dummies* books is that you can read the chapters in whatever order you want. Feel free to jump around and find the information most relevant to where you are right now. If you're totally new to smoothies, then start with Chapter 1 to get the basics first; if you're not sure whether that blender hiding in the depths of your kitchen cabinet is up to the task of smoothie creation, head to Chapter 2 to check out your equipment options. If you're already making smoothies but want tips on how to shop and prepare your ingredients, Chapter 3 is for you. For details on what ingredients to use, including greens, fruits, superfoods, and liquids, head over to Part II. Experienced smoothie drinkers may go to Parts III and IV for plenty of great healthy recipes. If you're looking to do a detox with green smoothies, check out Chapter 16.

Not sure where to begin? Sit back, relax, and start with Part I. It outlines the most important health benefits of green smoothies and what changes you can expect to see and feel from drinking them every day.

I feel blessed and honored to share my knowledge and experience with you. No matter what your starting point or health goal is, I wish you great success and many delicious green smoothies ahead!

Part I
Getting Started with Green Smoothies

getting started
with

Green
Smoothies

In this part . . .

- ✔ Discover the nutritional benefits of dark leafy greens and understand why they're such an essential food in a healthy, balanced diet.

- ✔ Get started with green smoothie basics, including juicing versus blending and why blending your greens is the best way to consume them.

- ✔ Explore your health potential by simply drinking one green smoothie every day.

- ✔ Consider whether your blender is up to the task of making smoothies and find out what features to look for if you're shopping around.

- ✔ Pick up tips on shopping for the best ingredients and how to wash and store your produce so it's always smoothie-ready.

Chapter 1

Reaping the Benefits of Green Smoothies

*W*hat exactly about leafy greens makes them such an important food for health? This chapter explores how you can boost your immunity, strengthen nails and hair, improve your digestion, sharpen your memory, lose weight, and even slow down or reverse certain diseases simply by drinking a green smoothie every day. With the information in this chapter, you'll be an expert and feel even more motivated to start blending up your own green smoothies.

Understanding the Nutritional Value of a Green Smoothie

Telling yourself to drink a green smoothie every day because you're "supposed to" isn't a great motivational tool, but knowing more about the nutritional value of greens increases your chances of keeping this new healthy habit in your diet for life. As an added bonus, you can also better explain your smoothie to family and friends when they see you drinking what they think is "green gunk" for the first time!

Chlorophyll: Drinking the green blood of plants

Plants, trees, leafy greens, and green vegetables are green because they contain a pigment known as *chlorophyll*. Plants use chlorophyll to absorb sunlight and change it into energy through a process called photosynthesis. One molecule of chlorophyll is very closely related in structure to one molecule of *hemoglobin* (human blood), so chlorophyll is sometimes referred to as the "blood of plants."

Because chlorophyll is so closely related to hemoglobin, when you ingest it, you're basically getting a free blood transfusion. Chlorophyll helps rebuild and replenish red blood cells almost instantly. When you eat green vegetables or leafy greens, you're actually ingesting edible energy from the sun, giving you an amazing, all-natural energy boost. Chlorophyll helps speed up healing and reduce risk of infection thanks to its antibacterial and antifungal properties. In addition, it protects against free radical damage. Chlorophyll also helps detoxify the lymph system, blood, and liver.

The pH factor: Getting alkaline

Maintaining an alkaline pH in the body is one of the best ways to prevent disease and stop premature aging. Ideally, your body's pH should be slightly alkaline, in the range of 7.365 to 7.385. When your pH is too high or too low, you can feel tired, gain weight, have poor digestion, suffer from skin breakouts, and feel aches and pains in your joints. Over time, an out-of-balance pH weakens your immune system, leaving you more at risk for viral and bacterial infections, including certain types of cancer.

Most food in the Standard American Diet (SAD) is highly acidic. Refined sugar, processed foods, meat, dairy, wheat products, alcohol, and coffee are all acid-forming. Stress alone can make you acidic, too. It should be no surprise that many people today are sick, tired, or both.

If you stay chronically acidic over several months or years, your body tries to correct itself toward alkalinity by leaching calcium from your bones to buffer the acid. Over the long term, that leaves you at higher risk of osteoarthritis and osteoporosis. Look at vegan animals in nature. They eat edible leafy greens as a dietary staple, and none of them suffer from loss of bone density later in life. Now, that's some (green) food for thought!

You don't have to give up all acidic foods, but the more alkaline foods you consume, the better your body can achieve a healthy pH balance. Leafy greens are one of the most alkaline-forming foods in nature. Just by adding more greens to your daily diet, you can counter the effects of other, high-acid foods in your diet.

Enjoying enzyme energy

Enzymes are tiny catalysts of energy that perform specific tasks in your body. Your body makes two main types of enzymes:

- *Metabolic enzymes* help grow new cells and repair old ones. A lack of metabolic enzymes can speed up the aging process, resulting in more wrinkles, bone loss, and aches and pains in the joints.
- *Digestive enzymes* assist with the digestion and assimilation of food — mainly proteins, carbohydrates, and fat.

You can help your body with its enzyme activities by bringing in more enzymes, either in food or supplement form. Food enzymes help digestive enzymes break down your food and help metabolic enzymes speed up your cellular repair. You find higher amounts of food enzymes in raw, uncooked fruits and vegetables. Most food enzymes are destroyed when you heat a food above 118 degrees Fahrenheit, so by consuming fresh fruits and uncooked leafy greens, your body gets the enzymes it needs naturally.

Calling fiber your friend

Without a doubt, fiber is the key for good digestive health. On average, Americans eat only 15 grams of fiber daily, yet the recommended daily allowance (RDA) is 38 grams per day for males and 25 grams per day for females (though the recommendations vary a bit depending on your age). What happens when your fiber intake is too low? Short-term, you can suffer from constipation and hemorrhoids. Long-term, a low fiber diet can increase your risk of heart disease, stroke, diabetes, and gastrointestinal problems.

Quickly increase your daily fiber consumption by drinking a green smoothie! Even better, add more fiber to your smoothie with two tablespoons of ground flaxseeds or chia seeds for an extra four to ten grams of fiber. Combining fresh whole fruits, leafy greens, and flax or chia gives you the perfect fiber-rich drink. All that extra fiber helps with weight loss by keeping you feeling full, prevents constipation, and enhances regularity.

Boosting your mineral intake

The noticeably bitter taste in leafy green vegetables comes from their high mineral content. In dark leafy green vegetables, you find plenty of calcium, iron, magnesium, zinc, manganese, phosphorous, and potassium. Just by adding a handful or two of leafy greens to your daily smoothie, you're getting a lot of extra minerals for very little effort.

The benefits of eating a mineral-rich diet include the following:

- ✔ Stronger teeth and bones, with a lower risk of osteoporosis
- ✔ Improved blood pressure
- ✔ Better muscle recovery after workouts
- ✔ Strengthened immune system
- ✔ Sharper memory and good brain function
- ✔ Thicker hair and stronger nails
- ✔ Clearer skin, fewer wrinkles, and a more youthful look
- ✔ Balanced thyroid function and hormonal system
- ✔ Stable blood sugar levels

Increasing vitamins for vitality

Your daily green smoothie offers a nutrient-dense health drink that's absolutely jam-packed with valuable vitamins for your health. In fresh fruits, you get vitamins A, C, E, and a whole array of disease-fighting antioxidants. In leafy greens, you get folate, vitamin B6, and vitamin K. Add some of the superfoods listed in Chapter 6 and you're boosting your vitamins even more. Now that's a great way to start the day!

Getting all the vitamins your body needs benefits your health by

- ✔ Fighting infections and boosting your immune system
- ✔ Helping heal wounds and reduce scarring
- ✔ Building strong bones and muscles
- ✔ Strengthening heart and red blood cells
- ✔ Improving the absorption of iron
- ✔ Increasing energy and vitality
- ✔ Strengthening eyesight
- ✔ Supporting kidneys
- ✔ Maintaining strong teeth and improving dental health
- ✔ Normalizing nerve function

Picking green protein

You may not think of spinach, spirulina, and kale as sources of protein, but they are! Greens are a natural powerhouse of protein, and they offer an easy-to-digest, high-fiber alternative to traditional animal-based options. Just think of horses, cows, water buffalo, giraffes, elephants, and gorillas; they're all huge muscle-mass animals, and they're all vegans! They get their protein from fresh, raw leafy greens.

Other plant-based proteins to add to your green smoothie include spirulina powder, hemp seeds, flaxseeds, chia seeds, tahini, fresh sprouts, and bee pollen. (Flip to Chapter 6 for important info on consuming bee pollen if you're allergic to bees or pollen.)

The benefits of eating more plant-based proteins include the following (many of which are benefits I cover in the preceding sections):

- ✔ Support an alkaline pH
- ✔ Don't raise cholesterol levels
- ✔ Encourage heart health
- ✔ Help strengthen the digestive tract
- ✔ Promote healthy bowel function
- ✔ Boast powerful anti-inflammatory effects
- ✔ Boost the immune system
- ✔ Reduce risk of metabolic syndrome
- ✔ Provide a rich source of minerals, vitamins, and antioxidants
- ✔ Contain high amounts of fiber
- ✔ Promote muscle recovery and repair
- ✔ Minimize aches and pains in the joints

Getting variety with greens

Wild animals instinctively practice variety in their eating habits, and they naturally move or graze from tree to bush to plant, eating small amounts of leaves from different sources. They do this to protect themselves from small amounts of toxins (called *phytotoxins*) in leaves that protect the plant from being overeaten.

When making green smoothies, the same rule of nature applies: Use variety in your greens. Buy different greens each week and practice rotating your greens every two to three days. (Chapter 4 gives a detailed list of what greens you can use.) Although you won't actually get sick from eating spinach, kale, or boy choy every day for months on end, those greens might not be as effective for you if you don't give them a break and switch them out every now and again. Another good reason to rotate your greens is to make sure you're not getting too much oxalic acid, especially if you have kidney disease (read more about that in Chapter 4).

To supplement or not to supplement

As you read through all the fantastic health benefits you can achieve from adding more nutrients to your diet, your first thought may be to skip the dietary changes and simply take a mineral and vitamin supplement. After all, isn't just taking a pill easier? That way, you know you're getting everything. In reality, your body doesn't absorb concentrated doses of nutrients from a small pill well. The fiber in food controls the pace at which the nutrients are absorbed. Because a multivitamin contains no fiber, it passes through your body very quickly, and you don't actually absorb most of the nutrients. You're left with little more than very expensive urine.

If you decide to supplement, choose only pure vitamins, also known as natural or whole food supplements, because these supplements are derived from actual whole food sources. (Most vitamins are made from chemicals and not real food sources.) Or better yet, stick with green smoothies and focus on getting plenty of real, whole fruits, vegetables, and leafy greens in your diet. Superfood powders are also a good option because they're whole foods dried and ground into powder form. *Note:* If you're a vegan or vegetarian, you need to take a B vitamin complex to cover your recommended daily nutritional needs for B12 and B6.

Smoothies versus Juice

This book focuses on green *smoothies*. What's the difference between a smoothie and a juice? A smoothie is made in a *blender*, where all the ingredients are blended with their fiber. Juice is made in a *juicer*, and that's a different appliance completely. A juicer separates the fiber from the liquid, creating a liquid juice with no fiber. To make green smoothies, you need a blender. (Refer to Chapter 2 to find out which blenders are best for making green smoothies.)

Toasting to a Healthier You

As the saying goes, "Your health isn't everything, but without your health, you have nothing." When you're healthy, you have more energy, you sleep better, you're naturally more motivated and inspired, you feel vibrant, you can handle stress better, and (most importantly) you can enjoy life. The biggest problem with living in the fast-paced modern world is that you can easily forget to take time for your health.

Appreciate your health now; treat your body like a temple by keeping it clean on the inside and out. Eat more foods high in nutrients, chlorophyll, fiber, and alkalinity to increase your chances of getting and staying healthy. It's a small investment that can benefit you and your family for many years to come. The following sections break down some of the health benefits of green smoothies.

Boosting immunity

Your best natural defense against illness is maintaining an alkaline pH, eating a diet high in fiber and nutrients, avoiding too many processed foods or chemical additives, and staying hydrated with plenty of water. Green smoothies check all these boxes in one fell swoop. Reducing stress, getting enough sleep, and exercising regularly definitely help, too.

One of the best ways you can support your immunity is to start before you get sick. Most people don't really think about what they're eating until they come down with something. Think of maintaining your health like you would maintain your car. If you schedule your car for regular maintenance, you're much less likely to deal with a breakdown later. The same goes for your body. Look at your green smoothie as a regular mini service check, boosting your body with valuable nutrients, antioxidants, chlorophyll, and fiber. If your body has all the tools it needs, more than often than not, it can fix itself.

Fighting fatigue

Processed foods, fried foods, heavy carbohydrates, and refined foods (such as white sugar and white flour) are *empty calories*. Not only are they difficult to digest, but they also provide very little in the way of nutrients for your health. Over time, eating a diet high in these foods leaves you at greater risk for nutritional deficiencies. Without the essential nutrients your body needs, you feel increasingly tired. Your internal organs are working overtime trying to survive off of economy fuel in a high-octane machine.

Giving your body a blended drink that's full of fiber, easy to digest, and loaded with vitamins, minerals, and chlorophyll is the best way to recharge your batteries and feel a natural boost of energy. When I drink my smoothie, I feel like I want to go for a walk and move! I never feel like I need to lie down and sleep. Not many people can say the same after eating a big pancake or waffle breakfast.

Living longer and better

For most people, the goal isn't just to live a long life but rather to live a long, happy, and healthy life. The only scientifically proven secret to longevity is *caloric restriction*. In other words, if you eat less over the course of several decades, you increase your chances of living longer. The Okinawans in Japan are often called the longest-living, healthiest people on the planet, living to more than 100 years old. They have a saying that translates to "Eat until 80 percent full." The problem with the fastest growing diseases today — heart disease and diabetes — is that they're both related to diets of excess and overeating.

Choose to invest time and effort into eating better foods now, and you'll benefit from the rewards for decades to come. A green smoothie gives you a nutrient-packed food without a lot of calories, helping reduce sugar cravings and control your appetite later. Eating better foods helps you feel satiated.

Improving memory

Sadly, dementia is no longer a condition affecting only older generations; symptoms are now showing up in folks as young as 45. Parkinson's disease is a progressive neurological disorder caused by a breakdown of cells in the part of the brain that produces a neurotransmitter called dopamine. The exact cause of Alzheimer's disease is still unknown, but it's shown to be related to chronic inflammation, nutritional deficiencies, toxicity, and raised cortisol levels from prolonged periods of stress. All these conditions have been linked to deficiencies in magnesium, vitamin D, selenium, omega-3 fatty acids, and B vitamins.

Thankfully, green smoothies give you plenty of magnesium in fresh leafy greens. (Your body needs magnesium in order to synthesize vitamin D.) Selenium occurs naturally in both Brazil nuts and walnuts. Add just one organic Brazil nut or three or four walnut halves to your smoothie to meet your recommended daily allowance of selenium. Omega-3s are readily available in both chia seeds and flaxseeds. And for all your B vitamins (especially B6 and B12), taking a B complex supplement is a good idea (see the sidebar "To supplement or not to supplement").

Strengthening digestion

You can improve your digestion for the entire day just by adding one green smoothie to what you currently eat daily. Drinking a large glass of green smoothie can easily double your fiber intake in an easy-to-digest blended form without a lot of added calories. I've had clients with digestive issues such as colitis, irritable bowel syndrome (IBS), leaky gut syndrome, chronic constipation, and even frequent or loose stool all see improvement in their conditions just by adding a green smoothie to their current diets.

Losing weight naturally

Strict, extreme diets may give you short-term results, but they aren't sustainable in the long run and don't promote lasting health. Many diets cut out fat and/or carbs, but a no-fat diet isn't good for your brain. In fact, omega-3 fatty acids are essential for proper brain function. And a no-carb diet can weaken digestion, leaving you constipated and suffering from bad breath (a sign of internal toxicity).

The only way to lose weight and keep it off is to

✔ Eat more nutrient-dense, high-fiber food and fewer empty calories.

✔ Exercise not only to burn fat but also to increase your resting metabolism.

Drink a daily green smoothie, and you've got the first point covered easily! Add some exercise into your routine, and just like that, you've found the best lifestyle combo for achieving and maintaining weight loss.

To jump-start your weight loss and get some motivation in your veins, try a three-day green smoothie detox. From there, you can make more changes, adding exercise and continuing to improve other areas of your diet. Refer to Chapter 16 for more information on detoxing with green smoothies, and check out Chapter 12 for green smoothie recipes that can help with weight loss.

A green smoothie is a fantastic replacement meal for losing weight. Make a commitment to yourself to do swap in a green smoothie at mealtime for 7, 14, 30, or even 60 days — whatever feels best for you. During that time, choose one meal per day — breakfast, lunch, or dinner — to replace with a green smoothie. Be sure to drink enough so you feel satisfied, anywhere from one-half to one liter of smoothie at a time.

Radiating Beauty from the Inside Out

Because fresh greens and fruits are so high in antioxidants, they naturally help with cell repair. Although that process starts on the inside, you can and will see the results on the outside. As you drink more green smoothies, you may start to notice improvements in your skin, stronger nails, brighter eyes, or thicker hair.

Your teeth may whiten, your gums may look healthier, and your breath may improve. These responses to such a small change in your diet are a sign that your diet was lacking in certain minerals or vitamins before.

Improving your skin

After my first three months of drinking green smoothies every day, a woman approached me in public and said, "Excuse me, but I just had to tell you that you have such beautiful skin." Before that, I'd *never* had anyone tell me that in my entire life! Now, it's a compliment I receive all the time. My reply is always, "Thank you, but it's coming from the inside. My skin looks good thanks to what I eat."

People are always surprised when I tell them that food is the key to natural beauty. Good skin comes from the inside; it has everything to do with what you eat or don't eat. Real beauty secrets aren't waiting for you in a cream or potion. The secret is on your plate and in your glass.

Diets high in fried foods, processed foods, and foods with refined sugar wreak havoc on your skin. Free radical damage from those foods to your cells speeds up the aging process and contributes to breakouts, oily skin, rashes, and wrinkles.

On the flip side, eating more whole food in its natural form repairs cellular damage from inside. Natural antioxidants in fruits, greens, and superfoods reduce free radical damage and slow down the effects of aging. The water in your smoothie adds extra hydration, which is always helpful for clearer skin, and the chlorophyll from leafy greens gives your skin a healthy glow.

Several years ago, I was covered from head-to-toe in a horrible, itchy rash that was diagnosed by doctors as everything from eczema to psoriasis to depression. I was desperate to hide my condition because it was especially bad on my face. I tried every single cream on the market for two years until I finally started to look at my diet. After making significant changes and adding green smoothies as a staple food, my skin started to clear on its own. Today, my skin is perfectly clear. I'm living proof that when you change your diet for the better, your skin changes for the better, too.

Reversing gray hair

Is it really possible to reverse gray hair just by drinking green smoothies?? Ann Wigmore says yes! She was actually the original inventor of the green smoothie, a renowned nutritionist and health practitioner and co-founder of the Hippocrates Health Institute in Florida and Puerto Rico. In the 1970s, she started making green smoothies, calling them her "energy soup." At that time, she was already in her 50s and had a full head of gray hair. Over time, as she drank lots of raw, uncooked leafy greens every day, she noticed that her gray hair started returning to its natural brown color! In fact, in her 80s, she had a full head of brown hair. She even had her students send a sample of her hair to a laboratory to prove that she wasn't using any chemical dyes. Her theory: Gray hair is linked to mineral deficiencies. Boost your diet with plenty of minerals, and the natural color will start to reappear.

In my personal experience, I've witnessed my hair become darker, thicker, shinier, and even curlier after changing to a plant-based diet and drinking green smoothies every day.

Strengthening nails

If you suffer from brittle nails or have ridges in your nails, it's time to start drinking your way back to health. The mineral that you need the most for strong nails (and hair) is *silicon* (not to be confused with artificial silicone). Silicon is found on the skins of fruits and also in seeds.

Chop up an apple or pear with the skin and add flax, chia, sunflower, or hemp seeds to your smoothie. In just a few weeks, you'll start to see and feel improvement in your nails.

Brightening eyes

I like to say that your eyes are the windows to your health. Did you ever see someone with drooping eyelids; dark under-eye circles; or eyes that appeared tired, bloodshot, or glassy? When you're deficient in minerals, overloaded with free radical damage, constipated, dehydrated, or not eating a high-fiber diet, your eyes are definitely going to show it.

When you're clean inside, your eyes become naturally brighter, more engaging, and vibrant. A high-antioxidant diet helps strengthen and repair your liver, and that helps minimize dark circles under the eyes and can even improve your eyesight. A high-fiber diet can reduce redness in the whites of the eyes. Eliminating refined sugar and processed foods and focusing on natural, whole, and pure foods helps tighten the upper eyelids, reducing droopiness and any glassy effect.

Tackling the Effects of and Risks for Various Maladies

If you or someone you love is suffering from an illness, use the nutrients, fiber, and chlorophyll in green smoothies to help naturally support a return to health. Green smoothies can help speed up your recovery time, rebuild your immune system, reduce pain, minimize inflammation, replenish your energy and vitality, strengthen your digestive system, and regulate blood sugars.

If you have any history of disease in your family, focus on green smoothie recipes to strengthen your body's natural inherent weakness. For example, if cancer runs in your family, include a green smoothie designed for fighting inflammation (see Chapter 13) in your diet two to three times a week. That way, you're actively working toward prevention. When you create a healthy lifestyle that includes regular exercise, reduced alcohol consumption, and nutrient-dense, fiber-rich foods (and cuts out smoking and excess stress), you're increasing your chances of living a very long, happy, healthy life.

Green smoothies complement any treatment or therapy, but inform your doctors of any significant changes you make to your diet while under their care.

Heart disease

The most significant risk factors of heart disease and stroke are an unhealthy diet and physical inactivity. To minimize your chance of developing cardiovascular disease, reduce your intake of foods that are high in salt, sugar, and unhealthy fat. Increase your exercise, eat healthy foods, and avoid smoking tobacco products. Maintain a healthy body weight. Choose a diet high in fruits and veggies; it's the best protection for your heart.

If you already suffer from cardiovascular disease, you can still make practical changes to your diet to slow down and, in some cases, even reverse your condition. As I note earlier in the chapter, the chlorophyll in greens has amazing positive effects on your blood cells. Greens also contain potassium, an important mineral for heart health. You can find recipes targeted at reducing risk of heart disease and managing symptoms in Chapter 13.

Diabetes

When can a blended drink made of fruits and greens be good for diabetics? When it's altered to suit blood sugar sensitivities. Safe fruit choices for diabetics include low glycemic index fruits such as grapefruit; fresh berries; and savory fruits such as cucumber, tomato, avocado, and bell pepper. (The *glycemic index* is a system that measures how a given food affects your blood sugar; lower numbers are better for diabetics.) Adding fiber in the form of flax-seeds or chia seeds helps stabilize blood sugars. Leafy greens are an excellent food choice for diabetics because they're high in minerals and fiber and have no negative effects on blood sugar levels.

If you're pre-diabetic, use green smoothies to help minimize your sugar cravings and get added fiber in your diet (the best defense against diabetes). If you're already diabetic, choose green smoothie recipes that are low in sweet fruits, such as the smoothies listed in Chapter 13. Use stevia powder to sweeten your smoothie without any ill effects on your blood sugar levels.

Cancer

Whether you're trying to prevent cancer, actively fighting it, or recovering from treatment, you should be focusing on reducing inflammation. Decreasing (but not eliminating) your intake of inflammatory foods automatically puts you on an anti-cancer diet. I'm talking about refined sugar, alcohol, processed foods, fried foods, meat, dairy, and wheat.

At the same time, increase your intake of anti-inflammatory foods such as fresh ginger, turmeric, fennel, and all dark leafy greens. Green smoothies are a great anti-cancer food because they're full of fresh and all-natural ingredients. Especially if you don't normally cook with turmeric or fennel, drinking green smoothies is an easy way to add these healing foods to your diet.

Fresh fruits and superfoods like acai powder, goji berries, or pome-granate powder are naturally high in antioxidants, an important element in food that helps build the immune system; fight disease; and repair from surgery, chemotherapy, or radiation. Leafy greens contain chlorophyll, which helps speed up the recovery process and boost your mineral reserve. You can find recipes targeted to your health needs after surgery, chemo, or radiation in Chapter 13.

Autoimmune disorders

Autoimmune diseases are conditions where the body's immune system starts attacking its own tissues rather than only foreign invaders such as viruses and bacteria. The most common autoimmune disorders are rheumatoid arthritis, lupus, multiple sclerosis, inflammatory bowel disease, Type-1 diabetes, hypothyroidism, and psoriasis. Although why these conditions happen or how exactly to stop the immune-attacking overdrive is still unknown, it's widely accepted that reducing inflammation helps significantly minimize symptoms, especially for pain and swelling in the joints.

 If you suffer from an autoimmune disorder, focus on an anti-inflammatory diet to help ease your symptoms. Your diet should be high in the following elements, all of which are easy to get in one green smoothie per day:

- ✔ Omega-3 fatty acids (naturally found in chia seeds, walnuts, and flaxseeds)

- ✔ Thirty-five to 40 grams of fiber daily (naturally found in fruit and vegetables)

- ✔ A *rainbow* of colors in your fruits and veggies, especially berries, yellow and red fruits, and dark leafy greens, all high in antioxidants

- ✔ Vitamins and minerals, especially vitamins C and E, calcium, and selenium

- ✔ Natural anti-inflammatory foods such as ginger, turmeric, and fennel

Anxiety and depression

Depression and anxiety can impact individuals of any age. The causes of each are rather complicated, and certainly, drinking a green smoothie isn't a fast fix for a serious psychological condition. However, diet can play a role in how much or how frequently you suffer.

Reducing your consumption of *bad mood foods* such as gluten, refined sugar, refined carbohydrates, and fried foods can help relieve the intensity of your symptoms. Increasing consumption of important brain nutrients such as omega-3 fatty acids, B vitamins, and selenium is important to stabilize brain function. By balancing your blood sugars throughout the day, you reduce the risk of mood swings.

Having a daily green smoothie creates a stable foundation for a healthy routine if you suffer from anxiety or depression. Include high-antioxidant foods and superfoods such as blueberries, goji berries, pomegranate, and acai powder to help improve brain health and nervous system function. Add ingredients that help balance blood sugars, such as grapes, coconut oil, avocado, fresh berries, and plenty of dark leafy greens. Use maca powder as a natural mood enhancer.

Chapter 2

Choosing the Best Equipment for Green Smoothies

In This Chapter

▶ Knowing what to look for in a blender

▶ Taking steps to avoid burning out a blender's motor

▶ Selecting a smoothie storage container

▶ Contemplating adding a juicer to your appliance family

*S*hopping for a new blender can be exciting and overwhelming at the same time thanks to the variety of brands and models available. In this chapter, I explain all the features you should look for in a blender. I highlight some of the most popular models available and offer some comparisons to make finding a blender that easily meets your needs and budget.

After you've chosen a blender and started making green smoothies, cleaning your blender and storing your smoothies are the next order of business. I give you easy instructions for those tasks in this chapter, too. And in case you decide to branch out into making green juices, I give you brief overview of juicing and how it compares to smoothies.

Picking a Blender

If you already have a blender, you can start making green smoothies right away. If not, you need to get a blender. The blenders I list here range from less than $50 to more than $400, but they've all been field-tested and can easily make a nice green smoothie. Keep in mind that using a standard household blender to make green smoothies is more than okay. The key is to make a smoothie and do the best you can. The following sections outline the important criteria to consider when you're shopping for a green smoothie blender.

Thinking about blender type

Your basic blender types include the following:

- ✔ **Professional/high-power:** These industrial-kitchen-strength blenders are the top of the line blenders with the highest available motor speed (up to 3 horsepower). You may have to go online or to a specialty appliance store to get them, but if money is no object and you're looking for the best blender that will feed an army and still keep going, stick to this category.

- ✔ **Household standard blender:** This group includes the classic, affordable kitchen appliance brands that you find in most stores. The pitcher size and motors vary, but overall these blenders are very good for green smoothies.

- ✔ **Immersion blender:** Also known as a *stick blender,* an *immersion blender* is a single shaft blender that you immerse in the ingredients. The immersion blender's motor usually can't blend fibrous green leaves, so it's not a good option for green smoothies.

- ✔ **Bullet blender:** The *bullet blender* is a small container that twists on top of the base. The smaller blender container makes adding large green leaves difficult and doesn't lend itself to multiple servings. For green smoothies, bullet blenders are simply too small and not the best option.

In the following sections, I give you more detail on the best two options for making green smoothies: the professional high-power blenders and standard household models.

Professional or high-power blenders

A *high-power blender* is any blender with a motor of 2 horsepower or above. These blenders are often used in commercial kitchens because they can withstand a lot of use. These models come with a higher price tag, but you also get a better warranty, improved customer service, and a more efficient motor. Here are some common brands:

- ✔ **Vitamix:** In the world of smoothies, Vitamix is the holy grail of blenders. Its top-selling 5200 blender has a 2 horsepower motor and offers a variable speed dial. It comes with a 64-ounce pitcher and a unique plunger that helps you safely move ingredients while blending. Unlike some other brands, this model doesn't have any preset buttons or timer features. It's a solid choice for making green smoothies.

- ✔ **Blendtec:** Blendtec is a popular commercial blender that you often see behind the counter in well-known coffee shops and smoothie bars. Its machine is fast, efficient, and well engineered for heavy use. The Blendtec Designer Series WildSide offers a sleek, absolutely gorgeous 3 horsepower blender with a unique digital display; it fits perfectly with a modern, clean kitchen design. Speaking of fit, the Blendtec sits at about 15 inches tall, making it easy to stash away under a cabinet on your kitchen counter. The Designer blender also has a nice range of preset buttons (for green smoothies, use the 40-second *smoothie preset*).

✔ **Omega:** The Omega BL630 blender is sometimes referred to as the "monster truck of blenders" — it has a huge base, a very large 64-ounce pitcher, and a 3 horsepower motor. This blender can blend anything! Plan on having a lot of counter real estate for this machine, though, because it's big! My favorite feature of the Omega is the timer function that allows you to set the blending time from 15 seconds up to 6 minutes. For a large family making a lot of smoothies, the Omega is the perfect choice.

✔ **Ninja:** Ninja offers a wide range of blender models at affordable prices. The 2.5 horsepower Ultima blender is putting some serious competition in the high-power blender market. Ninja actually has two stacks of very sharp blades, one at the bottom and one in the middle of the pitcher shaft, making it a sheer powerhouse in terms of getting a nice, smooth blend. The Ninja Ultima is a very good blender at almost half of the price of its 2 horsepower and 3 horsepower competitors. If you're looking to spend more than you would for a standard blender but can't afford the top of the line, the Ninja is a great choice for you.

Reliable names in household blenders

Standard household blenders are a fine, affordable option for green smoothie making. Popular brands include the following:

✔ **Kitchen Aid:** As a trusted household name in kitchen appliances, Kitchen Aid offers a classic blender at a reasonable price with its Diamond Vortex 5-speed blender. With a 60-ounce container and an easy-to-read display for the five speeds, the Diamond Vortex is a good choice for making green smoothies.

✔ **Cuisinart:** Cuisinart offers a sleek blender suitable for green smoothies called the SmartPower Deluxe. This blender has a smaller (48-ounce) glass pitcher.

✔ **Hamilton Beach:** The Hamilton Beach Smoothie Smart is the most affordable of all the blenders I mention in this chapter. The 40-ounce glass pitcher has an easy-pour spout. With a very small investment, you can be making your first green smoothie in minutes!

Not panicking over price

Do you need to invest in the most expensive blender when you start making green smoothies? Not at all! Of course, you're going to enjoy a smoother drink from a pricier blender thanks to its better motor, but a standard household blender can still make a really great and very drinkable smoothie. Remember, you can drive a beautiful 6-cylinder engineered car or a basic 4-cylinder model, and you'll arrive at your destination either way. (The earlier section "Thinking about blender type" has the lowdown on household and high-power blenders.)

My advice: Start with the best blender that you can afford. Make your green smoothie every day. If you have a chance to upgrade later, do it. You can always sell your starter blender, or give it to a loved one to spur that person's healthy jump start. I've bought several different blenders over the years while traveling around the globe, and I never let having a cheaper model stop me from making a great smoothie. Now that I'm finally settled in one place, I'm happily enjoying a nicer blender, but that's a good eight years after I started making green smoothies! The most important thing is that you're still actually making (and drinking) green smoothies.

Looking for specific blender features

You're ready to take the plunge and buy a blender for making green smoothies. Even if you've narrowed down your choices according to price (see the preceding sections), you may be surprised to find a lot of competition for your blender dollars. To get the best blender for your needs, think about the important points in the following sections.

Motor speed

The main reason blenders can cost from $50 to $400+ has to do with the quality and speed of the motor that runs the blender. A standard household blender usually has 600 watts or 700 watts, which equates to a 0.8 or 0.9 horsepower motor. At the high end of blender motors are the 2, 2.5, and 3 horsepower models. To give you a comparison: A 0.9 horsepower motor blends at a max speed of about 150 miles per hour, a 2 horsepower motor at a speed of 240 miles per hour, and a 3 horsepower motor at a whopping 300 miles per hour.

What's the difference for your actual smoothie? A faster motor blends more smoothly. It breaks down the pieces of greens and fruit into miniscule pieces, and the blended result is more uniformly smooth. Higher horsepower motors are also more durable, have better warranties, and are usually rated at a professional quality grade.

Pitcher size and material

The pitcher size is the actual volume of liquid that your blender carafe or container holds. How many people are you making smoothies for each day? If it's just one or two people, any size pitcher will do. But if you're feeding a family bigger than that, a larger size (60 ounces or more) will better suit your needs.

The other important question when it comes to either type of pitcher is "Do you want that in glass or plastic?" In the old days, people shied away from plastic pitchers because of the lower-quality plastics and concerns over chemicals leaching into the food. BPA, or Bisphenol-A, is the hazardous component of the old polycarbonate plastic containers. Luckily, technology has since improved, and now most appliance companies offer BPA-free plastic pitchers for their blenders. If the blender you're looking at is plastic, look for "BPA-free" on the front of the box.

Even with the rise of BPA-free plastic, a lot of folks still prefer glass pitchers. It's definitely a matter of personal preference (I use both and am equally happy), but here are some points to consider:

- **You can put both glass and BPA-free plastic pitchers in the dishwasher.**
- **Glass pitchers are heavy.** Larger pitchers (60 ounces and over) are usually plastic simply because a glass version would be too heavy. But even more-moderately sized glass pitchers may be unwieldy for Junior or Grandpa to use safely.
- **Glass pitchers can break or chip more easily than plastic.** In fact, blenders with 2 horsepower or faster motors use plastic pitchers because their extreme high blending speeds could cause glass containers to break.
- **Because glass pitcher blenders are usually smaller, they fit well under the kitchen cabinet for easy storage.** Check out the later section "Location, location, location: Surveying your storage needs" for more on this consideration.

Blade safety

Especially for parents with young children, blade safety is an important issue. Most blenders have one metal blade that's tucked all the way in the bottom of the pitcher. (The exception to that is the Ninja blender, which has two sets of blades, as I note earlier in the chapter.)

Blendtec takes the prize for having the safest blender blade, using a special design with no sharp edges at all. The duller-style blades are designed to crush, mill, and cut while causing less damage to brushes, spoons, or utensils and keeping fingers safe during cleaning or wiping.

Keeping your blender clean

The best way to keep your blender clean is to rinse it immediately after each use. If you don't have time, at least fill the blender pitcher with water and let it sit in the sink until you have time to wash it later.

When you have a few minutes to really clean up, you can either put the pitcher in your dishwasher or wash it by hand. To manually clean your pitcher, here's what you can do:

1. **Rinse the pitcher with water and refill it about halfway with clean water.**

2. **Add a few drops of liquid dish detergent, 2 tablespoons of white vinegar, or the juice of half a lemon.**

   Add 1 to 2 teaspoons of baking soda as well if you're trying to remove the odor of raw garlic or turmeric.

3. **Secure the lid on the blender and pulse the motor a few times, slowly increasing the speed to high; blend at high speed for about 30 seconds.**

4. **Remove the water mixture and make a final rinse with clean water; place the pitcher upside on a dish drying rack or a towel and let air dry.**

Some pitchers — usually glass or smaller ones — have a piece that locks the blade into the pitcher. (Larger pitchers are typically all one piece.) If your blender is the kind that comes apart, give it an extra cleaning once a week. Take the pitcher apart, rinse any debris around the rubber gasket and the bottom of the blade, let dry, and gently secure the pieces back into place.

Regardless of the placement or number of blades, you can make any blade safer by being conscientious about how you clean and store it. I recommend you rinse the blades by hand and set them to dry on a towel far out of reach (I like to leave mine on top of the refrigerator). Don't put them in the dishwasher or leave them on a countertop if you have small children in the house.

Location, location, location: Surveying your storage needs

Most people forget about this point until after they get the blender home, but where you need to/can keep your new appliance is an important factor to consider when buying your blender. Do you plan to leave it on the counter so it's ready whenever you want a smoothie or stash it in a cabinet when you aren't using it? I prefer to leave my blender on the counter because experience tells me that if my blender is staring at me every day, I'm much more likely to actually use it. I'm not one to fuss with pulling appliances out.

Do you prefer to keep your other small appliances out or put them away after use? That may help you decide what works best for you.

Of course, your counter space and cabinet height may dictate whether you can store your chosen blender out in the open. Check out the real estate in your kitchen to see where your blender can actually fit. Most large blenders are too tall to fit between your counter and the cabinet above it, whereas a smaller blender can sit there perfectly. Even the interiors of some cabinets may not have enough space to accommodate the height of some blender pitchers. You can see a side-by-side size comparison of blenders in Figure 2-1. Especially if you're taking the plunge to buy an expensive blender, you want to think about these practicalities and take some measurements before heading to the store.

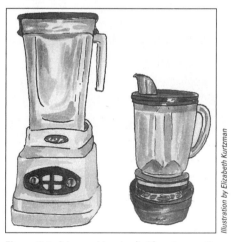

Illustration by Elizabeth Kurtzman

Figure 2-1: A larger blender (left) and a smaller household model (right).

Making Smoothies without Killing Your Blender

You've bought your first big bag of produce for smoothie making, and now you're ready to get home and start blending as fast as possible. You're thinking about all the healing power in those greens and can't wait to start drinking them in a blended, liquid form! You pull out the blender, add some greens and fruits, hit the blend button, and watch with great anticipation as your blender motor quickly blends, slows, groans, and dies.

I've been teaching green smoothie classes for almost ten years. The biggest mistake my students make is that in all the excitement of making their first smoothie, they forget to *add water*. Blending greens alone is totally possible in a 3 horsepower blender, but in a standard household blender, it's virtually impossible. In household blenders, you must add water before adding greens. Otherwise, the motor gets stressed trying to spin its blades on just greens, and it's kaput before you've even made your first green smoothie.

To avoid sending your blender to an early grave, follow these basic blending steps:

1. **Add chopped fruit and water first and secure the lid on the blender.**

2. **Blend, starting at a low speed and gradually increasing to high.**

3. **Stop blending; add your leafy greens and resecure the lid.**

4. **Blend again for 30 to 45 seconds until your drink is smooth.**

5. **Pour into glasses and serve.**

Congratulations! You now have a blender that can continue to serve you many healthy smoothies to come.

Storing Your Smoothies

If you like the idea of making your smoothie in advance and storing it in the fridge overnight, or if you'll drink half of your smoothie when you make it and the rest later in the day, you may be wondering how to best store it. The first thing you need is a proper container. I recommend a glass or BPA-free plastic vessel with a lid and a large, attached plastic straw. The lid helps keep the air out of your smoothie; too much exposure to air causes oxidation, which makes your smoothie go bad more quickly. The straw makes drinking your smoothie on the go easier. Green smoothies keep for up to 2 days when refrigerated in a sealed container.

Here are some other do's and don'ts for storing your smoothie:

- ✔ Don't leave your smoothie in the blender pitcher in the fridge; doing so leaves it vulnerable to air exposure and oxidation.

- ✔ Do fill your smoothie close to the top of the container (about ¼ to ½ inch) to reduce excess air space.

- ✔ Do clean your container with warm water and dish detergent, white vinegar, fresh lemon juice, and/or baking soda in between use.

Factoring Juicing into the Equation

People sometimes think green smoothies and green juices are basically the same thing, but they actually have some key differences. *Green juice* is made in a juicer, which separates the ingredients' fiber from their liquid; you drink only the liquid. A green smoothie, on the other hand, blends the fiber and liquid together in a blender, making a thicker drink that keeps all the fiber intact. The main focus of this book is on green smoothies. However, green juices are certainly great for your health too.

One of the major benefits of juicing is that you can get a much higher concentration of vitamins and minerals than what you could ever possibly eat in one sitting. Because all the fiber is removed, your body absorbs the nutrients in juice quickly. When you're sick or looking to boost your nutrition, having one green juice in addition to your green smoothie every day can help bring your body back to health more quickly. You can drink a fresh juice as a snack or with a meal. I personally make a green juice for breakfast and a green smoothie for lunch every day, and I love them both!

 If you're new to smoothies, my suggestion is stick with smoothies. Don't overwhelm yourself with the pressure of having to learn how to make juice, too. Over time, if you get more interested in expanding your culinary skills, you may want to get a juicer and start making juices.

Chapter 4 explains how to add fresh wheatgrass to a smoothie. If you're interested in juicing your own wheatgrass at home, you need a masticating juicer. The Omega 8004 is a great model for making fresh wheatgrass juice. Other options include the Champion juicer and the Hurom vertical slow-press juicer.

For more information on making fresh juice and ideas for different types of recipes, check out *Juicing & Smoothies For Dummies* by Pat Crocker (John Wiley & Sons, Inc.).

Chapter 3

Shopping and Preparing for Your Green Smoothies

. . . .

In This Chapter

▶ Focusing on fresh, organic ingredients (but knowing when compromise is okay)

▶ Breaking down the merits of fresh, frozen, canned, and dried foods

▶ Cleaning and storing your produce

. . . .

*W*ith high quality, fresh ingredients, you can make some seriously great-tasting smoothies that just happen to be great for your health, too. In this chapter, I explain where to buy your produce, how to find the freshest ingredients, and when to choose organic, and I give you tips for using frozen and dried fruits. I also tell you how to wash and store it all after you get those yummy fruits and greens home.

Knowing What to Look for in Smoothie Ingredients

Shopping for produce for green smoothies isn't difficult when you understand some basic principles of fresh food. When you know what to look for, your shopping experience is much easier and more efficient. Here's a good breakdown of what to look for in fresh fruits and leafy greens:

> ✔ **Keyword: fresh!** Nothing trumps the freshest-looking produce. Give those peaches a soft squeeze to make sure they're not too hard. Check the apples and pears for firmness. Look under the strawberry pack to make sure you don't see any mold. Leafy greens should be, you know, green, and not yellow or brown.

If you see an excessive amount of fruit flies hovering over a fresh fruit bin, take that as a sign that there's most likely rotten fruit somewhere in the bunch. You can safely choose fruit with just one or two fruit flies, but it's best to avoid fruits that are swarming with them.

✔ **Try to buy in season when possible.** Eating produce in season gives you the freshest possible food because chances are it hasn't had to travel across the world to get to your plate, or in this case, your blender. Even if it's not organic, it's still a good choice if it looks fresh!

✔ **Go green (for bananas).** Green bananas are actually a very practical buy if you only shop once a week. Buy three or four ripe bananas and three or four greens ones; that way, you have a few fresh ones for now and some that will be ready later in the week.

Debating organic versus non-organic

Organic food not only tastes better, but it's also better for you. Fewer chemicals sprayed on the fruits and veggies means they're less toxic to both you and the environment. And the higher-quality soil used in organic farming gives you more nutrients in the food. In an ideal world, I'd love to tell you to eat only 100-percent USDA certified organic food, but I know that financially that's just not realistic for most people. In a lot of places, you can't even find organic produce, or what you can find isn't that fresh.

First and foremost, know that buying organic doesn't have to be an all-or-nothing proposition. I personally buy about 60 to 70 percent of my food organic because that's what I have access to where I live, and I'm totally okay with it. Even if you buy 10 percent of your food organic, it's a start. Do what you can. A non-organic green smoothie is still better than no green smoothie at all!

Discover which fruits require fewer pesticides and are safer to buy non-organic and also which ones are most heavily sprayed by checking out the Environmental Working Group's Dirty Dozen and Clean Fifteen list of pesticide-heavy foods at www.ewg.org/foodnews/.

I talk more about produce shopping on a budget later in this chapter, but here are some tips specifically for buying organic on a budget:

✔ **Look for sales.** I love to cruise the organic produce section of the supermarket looking for bargains, and I usually find something on sale, especially leafy greens (perfect for a smoothie)! Just make sure that what you buy looks fresh. Don't sacrifice freshness for an organic label.

✔ **Buy in bulk.** Sometimes you can buy larger bags of, say, organic kale or apples at a cheaper price than the individual items.

✔ **Shop around.** Getting a feel for what prices are best takes a little time, but checking out different supermarkets and farmers' markets can really pay off. Eventually, you'll know exactly where to go for what and how much you should pay.

✔ **Join a local CSA.** A *community supported agriculture,* or CSA, is a community-based cooperative relationship connecting local farmers (growers) to customers (consumers). Hooking up with a CSA can be a great way to start getting more locally grown, organic food into your diet at an affordable price. Check out the nearby sidebar for more on CSAs.

✔ **Check online.** You can often find 100-percent certified organic spices and superfood powders at discounted rates online — sometimes with free shipping too!

Get to know your produce better with some simple sticker code detective work. Figure 3-1 outlines the difference between *price look up* (PLU) codes on fresh produce and what the code number means. The PLU code can help you identify whether or not your produce is organic or conventionally grown. ***Note:*** The PLU code for genetically modified (GMO) produce isn't currently mandatory, so don't expect to see that one often, if ever. For more information on GMO foods, refer to the "Avoiding genetically modified fruits and vegetables" section in this chapter.

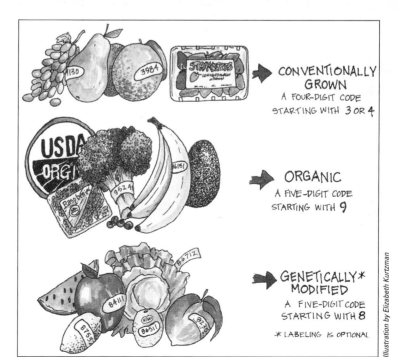

CONVENTIONALLY GROWN
A FOUR-DIGIT CODE STARTING WITH 3 OR 4

ORGANIC
A FIVE-DIGIT CODE STARTING WITH 9

GENETICALLY* MODIFIED
A FIVE-DIGIT CODE STARTING WITH 8
* LABELING IS OPTIONAL

Illustration by Elizabeth Kurtzman

Figure 3-1: The PLU codes provide valuable information.

Taking advantage of a local CSA

Community supported agriculture (CSA) is an easy and affordable way for you to buy locally grown and USDA certified organic food directly from the farmers. Here's how it works: Join a CSA and pay a weekly or monthly flat fee. Every week, you receive a box of freshly picked organic produce, delivered to your door or to a nearby pickup location. Some CSAs offer different box sizes to accommodate both single people and larger families. As the growing seasons change, you may receive different combinations of fruits and veggies. (Personally, I find that really fun because it gets me experimenting with new foods I may not usually buy, such as kohlrabi, parsnips, organic beets, and their greens.)

The benefits of buying from a CSA are twofold: You save time (and usually money) in shopping for your fresh, organic produce, and you help local farmers stay in business. A quick Internet search for "CSA + [your local area]" should point you to your local CSA options. You can also ask for information at your local health food store.

Putting your green into organic greens

If you can only afford to invest a small amount of your weekly budget in organic items, spend that money on organic leafy greens. Because greens have such a large surface area, they often get doused with pesticides. With organic greens, you're not only avoiding the chemical pesticides but also getting more minerals and nutrients in every leaf. Even buying half of your greens organic can make a difference! (Find out more about budgeting in the later section "Finding produce on a budget.")

Choosing organic spices

Try to buy 100-percent certified organic spices to avoid any added fillers or low quality ingredients. Look for organic spices on sale, either online or at the supermarket, and stock up then. One spice bottle can easily last two months; that makes it pretty affordable to buy on sale and save.

If you can get fresh ginger, use that instead of ground ginger (though you may want to keep ground ginger on hand a backup for times when you run out of fresh ginger).

Avoiding genetically modified fruits and vegetables

Several studies on genetically modified (GM or GMO) foods suggest consumption of GMOs may carry some health risks. Higher risk of food allergies; infertility; damage to the kidneys, liver, adrenal glands, spleen, and heart; weakening of the immune system; and reduction of brain size have all been linked to eating GMO foods. Clearly, more research needs to be done in order to understand the long-term effects to human health. In the meantime, avoiding GMOs as much as possible is definitely a good idea.

Other reasons to avoid GMO foods include the following:

- ✔ Large factory GMO farms sell mass-produced, non-organic food at such a low cost that small, local, organic farmers are unable to compete.

- ✔ All GMO seeds are patented, leading to a future of heavily controlled food pricing.

- ✔ GMO food crops require pesticides and can never be organically grown.

- ✔ GMO seeds that travel by wind can contaminate nearby organic farms and ecosystems (the future environmental implications of this issue are still uncertain).

- ✔ Large amounts of chemicals used in growing GMO foods harm local ecosystems and animal habitats.

Many countries have laws that require labeling of all GMO foods. In the United States, however, labeling of GMO foods isn't mandatory, although some states are actively fighting to change the current laws. If you want to join the citizens' petition to demand proper labeling of GMO foods in the United States, go to `http://truthinlabelingcoalition.org` or `http://act.thenhf.com/5948/us-gmo-foods-petition`.

Where does that leave you, the health-conscious consumer? By law, certified organic foods can't be genetically modified, so choosing all 100-percent USDA-certified organic products is the only way to avoid GMOs. Outside of organic foods, you can avoid products made from the two most commonly genetically modified foods grown in the United States today: soy and corn, including high fructose corn syrup (HFCS), soy milk, and tofu. Luckily, you're not using any of those ingredients in your green smoothies.

Buying Your Produce

Staying committed to making green smoothies is much easier when you have a plan. Ideally, you should shop for produce a few times a week to get the freshest ingredients possible. If that doesn't work for you time- or schedule-wise, at least make a plan to shop once a week.

When deciding where to buy your produce, first check out your options. Find out what stores are near you. Do you have supermarkets, health food stores, farmers' markets, or membership warehouse clubs? Where do you usually shop, and what's most convenient for you? Your normal supermarket stop is a good starting point for buying fruits and greens. It won't take long for you to figure out which store has the best apples and where to find organic kale.

Making a list

Especially if you're new to making green smoothies, start your shopping with an itemized list to make sure you don't forget any essentials. Decide which smoothies you plan to make with the goods from this shopping trip and write down the main ingredients for each one, noting how many servings you need.

Head to www.dummies.com/extras/greensmoothies for a shopping list that can help you get started when purchasing ingredients for your green smoothies.

Use your list as a guide, but not as something set in stone. If you need peaches for example, and they're too expensive or don't look fresh, don't hesitate to find a suitable replacement, such as kiwis or pears.

Over time, as you become familiar with the best green smoothie ingredients and have a better idea of what fruits and greens you can find in your area, you probably won't need any list at all. But I must admit, even after years of making green smoothies, I still occasionally forget the bananas! And when that happens, I add more apples, pears, oranges, or persimmons.

Starting with local farmers' markets

Your local farmers' market is the best place to find the freshest (and often cheapest) smoothie ingredients. Depending on where you live, your farmers' market may only be open in spring, summer, and/or fall, but even having access to local and fresh ingredients for part of the year is a plus.

The benefits of eating locally grown food include

- ✔ The reduced transportation time from farm to blender gives you fresher food.
- ✔ Eating locally grown food can help reduce your risk of seasonal allergies.
- ✔ Choosing different seasonal foods local to your area helps to keep variety in your diet.

> ✔ Longer transport times increase the risk of bacterial contamination in foods.

Know, though, that not everything you find at a farmers' market is local, organic, and/or cheaper than store prices. Check the labels before you buy, and look for signs that say "locally grown." If you're unsure, don't be afraid to ask a staff member or vendor.

Look for the following smoothie essentials at your farmers' market when they're in season:

> ✔ Locally grown leafy greens such as dandelion greens, kale, Swiss chard, arugula, or romaine lettuce
>
> ✔ Fresh peaches, nectarines, and plums
>
> ✔ Locally grown apples and pears
>
> ✔ Watermelon, strawberries, and blueberries
>
> ✔ Fresh local oranges (for people in warmer climates)

Search for sale bins in the back of the farmers' market. They often sell fruits that are fresh but slightly bruised or imperfect and greens that are one or two days old at half the price! If you cut away the bruised parts, you've still got perfect fruits for a smoothie. Soak day-old greens in water for 20 minutes and rinse them to help bring them back to life.

If you don't know where to find your local farmers' market or whether you even have one, ask around. Inquire at your local health food store or in your supermarket. Scan notice boards for flyers or postings. Check your local paper in the community events section. You can also search online at `www.localharvest.org/farmers-markets`.

Finding produce on a budget

Eating healthy on a budget is definitely possible with just a little bit of planning and effort. Approach your food shopping with the same savvy that you use to buy clothes, personal items, or household goods. On any given week, the smoothies you make may be determined by what's on sale at the supermarket, and that's okay!

Here are some tips for smart smoothie shopping on a budget:

> ✔ **Shop around.** You may have to go to more than one store to get the best prices.
>
> ✔ **Be flexible.** Replace ingredients to accommodate what you can afford or what's on sale. For example, if fresh mango is too expensive, use nectarines or grapes instead.

✔ **Join a membership warehouse club.** Especially if you're shopping for a large family, buying fresh ingredients in bulk at a membership-only supermarket can really pay off in the long run.

✔ **Stay committed.** If you're on strict budget, don't give up just because you can't achieve the ideal plan right now. Buy what your budget allows. Even having two or three green smoothies a week makes a big difference in your health!

Thinking about fresh versus frozen

Frozen produce can be really tempting when you want an ingredient that's not in season, but ultimately, your best choice for smoothie ingredients is fresh. Fresh and uncooked fruits and veggies are in their most natural state. In a raw form, all the enzymes that provide extra energy for digesting and absorbing your food remain intact.

Think of it this way: If you put a bunch of freshly picked spinach in water, you may notice the leaves turning to face the sunlight in your window after several minutes. That's a remarkable sign that those greens are still a live food. Take those same greens and freeze them, and you've destroyed the live enzymes, rendering the food dead. You're a live being, so eating more live foods brings you to a higher state of health.

Depending on where you live, though, you may not have access to fresh produce in the winter. If that's the case, you can certainly supplement your winter green smoothies with store-bought frozen leafy greens or berries, knowing that you're doing the best you can with what's available. Choose flash frozen foods, which have the least processing, and check the labels to make sure the products have no added salt or sugar. (Frozen greens can have added salt, and frozen fruits often contain added sugar). In warmer months, go back to buying fresh (and hopefully more local) ingredients.

Freezing fresh fruits is a practical way to stock up on sale items or prepare in advance for the first few months of winter. Look for two-for-one sales on berry packages and great deals on bananas. You can save super ripe sale fruits such as peaches, grapes, plums, apricots, and even watermelon from going overripe by cutting away any bruised or brown parts before freezing. Head to the later section "Freezing" for full instructions on how to prepare fruits for freezing.

Considering canned and dried options

Canned foods are definitely the least preferred option for making healthy smoothies. Canned greens (such as spinach, collard greens, or mustard greens) almost always contain high amounts of added salt, and canned fruit is usually packaged in sugar-filled syrup. Even no-sugar-added versions can be problematic because the aluminum in the cans themselves can leach into the food. (Aluminum poisoning has been directly linked to a higher risk of Parkinson's and Alzheimer's disease.) Canned food isn't fresh, and those added ingredients don't offer anything for your health.

Dried fruit is a more acceptable option, but you do have to consider a few points. On one hand, dried fruits have more sugar than fresh fruit because the drying process concentrates the natural sugars. Non-organic dried fruit is heavily preserved with sulfites, which have been linked to higher rates of asthma, especially in children.

On the other hand, organic dried figs, prunes, dried dates, or raisins can serve as a delicious natural sweetener in smoothies, especially when you're using bitter greens. Organic dried apricots and cherries can offer a great source of natural iron. Dried fruits maintain their freshness for a few months, so they're a convenient replacement and/or supplement to fresh fruits in winter months.

When using dried fruits in smoothies, keep the following guidelines in mind:

- ✔ Choose organic options to avoid preservatives such as sulfites.

- ✔ Because of the higher sugar concentration, dried fruits aren't recommended for diabetics. Anyone trying to lose weight should use dried fruits minimally.

- ✔ Rehydrate raisins and dried cherries by soaking them in 1 cup of water overnight. Rinse with fresh water and then add the fruit to the blender. Rehydrating dried fruits opens up their natural flavor and helps to create a smoother texture in the smoothie.

- ✔ Avoid using tropical dried fruits in your smoothies. Dried papaya, pineapple, and coconut often contain added sugar (sometimes manufacturers even dip the fruit in sugar before drying).

Caring for and Prepping Your Produce

Buying fresh fruits and greens is the first step in making a successful smoothie. But what do you do with everything after you've got it home? Taking a few minutes to wash and store your produce properly can save you time later and help keep everything fresh. In the following sections, I give you the lowdown on cleaning, keeping, and freezing your fresh green smoothie ingredients.

Washing

Get in the habit of washing all fruits and veggies as soon as you get home, before putting anything in the fridge. That way, you know that everything's been cleaned, and you don't have to think about it again later. Wash organic produce separately from non-organic.

Follow these steps to wash your produce (see Figure 3-2):

1. **Designate a large plastic tub just for washing produce.**

   Depending on the size of your household and how much produce you buy, you may need a tub anywhere from five to ten gallons in size. Don't use this tub for household cleaning, painting, or any other chemical projects.

2. **Fill your cleaning tub with room temperature or slightly cool tap water; add 1 tablespoon of white vinegar for every gallon of water.**

3. **Let the veggies soak in the water and vinegar mix for 10 minutes.**

4. **Gently pour the water and produce into a colander (for big shopping trips, you may need two or three large colanders).**

   Rinse thoroughly with tap water and allow to air dry for up to 30 minutes.

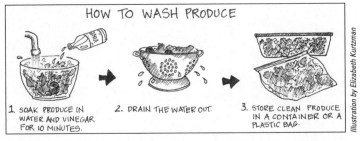

HOW TO WASH PRODUCE

1. SOAK PRODUCE IN WATER AND VINEGAR FOR 10 MINUTES.

2. DRAIN THE WATER OUT.

3. STORE CLEAN PRODUCE IN A CONTAINER OR A PLASTIC BAG.

Illustration by Elizabeth Kurtzman

Figure 3-2: Properly wash and store your produce when you get it home.

Storing

You can put clean fruit and veggies directly in your refrigerator bins. Greens require a bit more protection, though. After washing leafy greens (see the preceding section), put them in plastic bags or plastic or glass containers with lids to store in the fridge. Minimizing exposure to air keeps greens fresh longer, so seal or wrap plastic bags tightly to keep the air out.

As you buy new produce, check the old items still in the fridge. Discard any moldy or wilted produce. If you have old fruit that feels soft but still looks ripe and edible, you can freeze it for later use as I outline in the following section.

Freezing

In the earlier section "Thinking about fresh versus frozen," I explain when freezing fruits is a good option and which fruits are best to freeze. When you're ready to freeze your fresh fruits, here's what you do:

1. **Wash and rinse the fruit as described in the earlier section "Washing."**

2. **Remove bits you won't want to put in a smoothie.**

   Cut away any stems, cores, or stones/pits. Peel bananas.

3. **Cut the fruit into small-to-medium pieces.**

4. **Place the fruit in plastic freezer bags; mark the date on the bags and put them in the freezer.**

   Use the fruit within three months of storage.

Avoid freezing raw tomatoes, bell peppers, cucumbers, or avocados; they simply don't taste very good when frozen and blended.

Part II
Making Your Green Smoothie Taste Great

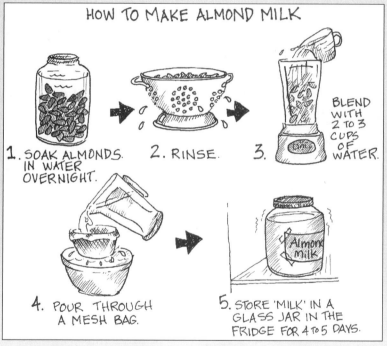

HOW TO MAKE ALMOND MILK

1. SOAK ALMONDS IN WATER OVERNIGHT.

2. RINSE.

3. BLEND WITH 2 TO 3 CUPS OF WATER.

4. POUR THROUGH A MESH BAG.

5. STORE 'MILK' IN A GLASS JAR IN THE FRIDGE FOR 4 TO 5 DAYS.

Illustration by Elizabeth Kurtzman

Green smoothies are easy to make, but just to be safe, visit www.dummies.com/extras/greensmoothies to make sure you avoid some common missteps.

In this part . . .

- ✔ Get the most out of your green smoothies by putting in the best leafy greens, fruits, and superfoods and leaving out some other ingredients.

- ✔ Know when to use powdered greens instead of fresh, what kind to use, and how much you need to add.

- ✔ Find out what superfoods are, how to use them in your smoothies, and which ones you need to achieve your health goals.

- ✔ Discover extra ingredients to add to smoothies to help you heal from common ailments like cold, flu, upset stomach, and headaches.

- ✔ Check out the top tips for making your smoothie taste great and how to adjust to flavor to get it just right if it's too bitter, too thick, or too sweet.

Chapter 4

Choosing Your Greens

In This Chapter

▶ Understanding the value of using (a variety of) greens

▶ Knowing which leafy greens are best for which purposes

▶ Exploring the powdered greens option

▶ Working with wheatgrass in smoothies

_I_f you thought you could only use spinach or kale in green smoothies, this chapter is definitely for you! Knowing what greens to add to your green smoothies gives you more confidence to actually go to the supermarket and pick up new and unusual items that perhaps you've never bought before. Using different greens is a great way to keep your smoothies interesting, find out more about the amazing healing elements in food, and understand how to best combine fruits and greens for your own personal taste. That knowledge helps you create new healthy habits for life.

In this chapter, I outline the most common leafy greens, herbs, and lettuces used in green smoothies, highlighting the health benefits of each. I address how and when to use green powders rather than fresh greens and give you some pointers on adding wheatgrass for an extra nutritional boost.

Getting the Lowdown on Adding Greens

Fresh leafy greens are really the flagship ingredient in green smoothies. Without them, you've still got a healthy, fiber-filled smoothie — and that's great — but you don't have the added minerals, chlorophyll, or healing power that greens bring to the party. Remember, a green smoothie has two main ingredients: fresh fruits and fresh greens. (Chapter 5 outlines what fruits to use in your smoothies.)

Leafy greens are a fantastic health food for many reasons, most notably the high vitamin and mineral content, antioxidants, and, yes, even protein. All leafy greens are low in calories. Combine that with the high fiber content, and greens become a great choice for balancing blood sugars and for weight loss. You can find more-detailed information on the nutrient content and healing power in leafy greens in Chapter 1.

Use variety in your greens, switching them out from time to time. Try not to use the same green for more than two weeks at a time to make sure that you don't get too many phytotoxins from any one type of green. *Phytotoxins* are naturally occurring in all leafy greens and are perfectly safe to eat, but keeping variety in your greens makes sure that you don't get too much. For more information on why, refer to Chapter 1.

If you're using a bitter green such as kale, you may want to stick with sweeter fruits such as pineapple, strawberries, pear, mango, papaya, or banana to help mask the bitter taste. Milder greens such as spinach or dandelion greens combine well with mild-tasting fruits such as kiwi or blueberries.

If you have certain thyroid conditions or kidney disease, you should use certain greens sparingly. Refer to the sidebar "Choosing greens when you have thyroid or kidney disease" in this chapter for more information, and talk to your doctor about your diet specifically.

Introducing the Top Greens for Health

Welcome to the world of dark, leafy edible greens! If you're not used to eating a lot of greens, this territory may be new and uncharted for you. But nearly all the green veggies I outline in this section are available in typical supermarkets. After just a few shopping trips, you'll be an expert at finding your fresh, leafy greens in the produce section. You may even start telling the checkout clerks which green is which as they look for the scanning codes or sharing your favorite smoothie recipe with other customers in line. After you start to reap all the benefits of green smoothies, you'll naturally want to share your new secret to success!

In the following sections, I list the most common greens used in green smoothies in order of popularity, starting with kale. *Note:* I'm assuming all these greens are in their natural, raw, and fresh state. For information on the differences among fresh, frozen, and canned ingredients, refer to Chapter 3.

When you hit the store and start choosing your own greens, keep the following points in mind:

- ✔ **Use variety!** Try to buy different kinds of leafy greens every week or couple of weeks, as I outline in Chapter 2.

- ✔ **Look for fresh, green-colored greens.** Avoid yellow, brown, or wilted leaves that look old.

- ✔ **Check the organic section for sales.** You can often find a good deal!

- ✔ **Use the recipes in Parts III and IV as a guide, but feel free to any alter recipe as needed.** Don't force yourself to buy Swiss chard if it looks brown around the edges, for example. Choose whatever greens look best (keeping variety in mind, of course).

- ✔ **Not all supermarkets carry the same stock of leafy greens.** For more access to different greens, you may have to shop at more than one place.

- ✔ **Ask the produce manager what day the store's greens are delivered.** Knowing what day to shop can be extremely useful to help you get the freshest greens.

- ✔ **Check out your local farmers' market.** Farmers' markets often have cheaper prices, and they may even have some locally grown options that bring in more variety for you, too.

Choosing greens when you have thyroid or kidney disease

Although balance and variety are the keys to success in eating a healthy diet, certain preexisting medical conditions may dictate which greens you eat and how often.

If you suffer from kidney disease or have only one kidney, you should minimize parsley and greens that are naturally high in oxalic acid, including spinach, Swiss chard, beet greens, kale, and collard greens. Your best choice of greens includes lettuce greens, bok choy, celery, and all other fresh herbs.

If you suffer from hypothyroidism, you should limit greens that contain high amounts of *glucosinolates,* naturally occurring elements in greens that can inhibit iodine uptake. Those greens include collard greens, mustard greens, kale, bok choy, and watercress. Focus on using lettuce greens, fresh herbs, dandelion greens, celery, alfalfa sprouts, and spinach instead. No matter what you're eating, having variety in your diet ensures that you're getting all the nutrients your body needs and not overdoing it with any one nutrient or food.

Kale

Kale has risen to the top of leafy green popularity in recent years, and it's certainly worthy of its superstar status. The large leaves of kale are a nutritional powerhouse, loaded with calcium, magnesium, vitamins A and C, folate, amino acids, and antioxidants. Kale's impressive concentration of nutrients helps boost your immune system, preventing many forms of cancer and other chronic diseases. The natural anti-inflammatory properties in kale can protect you from heart disease and atherosclerosis; the high fiber content lowers cholesterol; and the healthy balance of omega-3 and omega-6 fatty acids keeps your body strong, healthy, and beautiful from the inside out. It's also an excellent plant-based source of iron for vegans and vegetarians.

You can find kale in both large and small leaves and with curly or flat leaves. The most common varieties include green curly kale, red kale (which is actually more purple in color), and dinosaur kale. All varieties of kale tend be naturally bitter.

Spinach

Fresh spinach is another top pick in green smoothies for a few practical reasons:

- ✔ It's conveniently sold prewashed in bags, making it a fast and easy option. (Refer to the sidebar "Weighing the prewashed shortcut" for tips on using bagged spinach and other greens.)
- ✔ It's available in virtually every supermarket.
- ✔ It has a mild taste that's very suitable for green smoothies.

The powerful combination of antioxidants in spinach — including vitamins C and E, beta carotene, manganese, zinc, and selenium — helps prevent osteoporosis, atherosclerosis, and high blood pressure. The antioxidant lutein found in spinach helps protect your eyes from cataracts and prevent macular degeneration. A high amount of flavonoids give spinach its anti-cancer and anti-inflammatory benefits; high levels of vitamin A help prevent skin aging; and an abundance of vitamin K keeps bones strong.

You find fresh spinach in many varieties, including small (baby) leaves, medium, and large leaves. Any variety will work in your smoothies.

Weighing the prewashed shortcut

The convenience factor in buying prewashed bagged greens is admittedly hard to overlook. When you're really busy, what better way to get your greens than to grab a bag of precut, prewashed spinach, collard greens, or kale and go? I'm not against taking shortcuts, but knowing exactly what you're buying is important. Fresh leafy greens sold loose are always freshest, and fresh is definitely best. Greens sold in sealed plastic bags or containers are often sprayed with extra chemicals to keep them looking fresh. Some widespread outbreaks of gastrointestinal illness have stemmed from bacterial contamination in packaged greens.

Ultimately, I encourage you to buy whatever works best for you. If you do choose bagged greens, be sure to rinse them well with water even if the bag says they've already been washed. Always clean fresh loose greens prior to using them. For instructions on how to wash your fruits and greens, refer to Chapter 3.

Swiss chard

Like other leafy green vegetables, Swiss chard is a good source of calcium that helps strengthen bones and teeth. It contains vitamin K and magnesium, both of which are important for brain and bone health. Swiss chard is packed with lutein, the essential antioxidant for healthy eyesight. The high fiber, chlorophyll, and nutrient concentration in Swiss chard make it a natural anti-cancer food. It's also a great choice for diabetics thanks to the fiber and syringic acid, both of which help stabilize blood sugar levels. Disease-fighting antioxidants, including beta carotene, vitamin E, vitamin C, zinc, and quercetin, are abundant in the large leaves of Swiss chard.

You may find this leafy green with a red, white, yellow, or green stem. It can also be called silverbeet, strawberry spinach, or Roman kale. The taste is mildly bitter, making Swiss chard a natural choice for green smoothies.

Watercress

Hippocrates, the father of modern medicine, referred to the watercress plant as the "cure of cures." He even built his first clinic near a river so he could grow watercress to help treat his patients. Watercress is a good source of iodine and is rich in fiber, antioxidants, vitamin C, beta carotene, folate, potassium, calcium, phosphorous, and iron. In fact, it has more calcium than milk, more iron than spinach, and more vitamin C than oranges! That iron content means watercress is helpful in treating anemia.

Natural sulfur glycosides found in watercress have been shown to soothe chronic coughing and bronchitis. Watercress is often recommended to alleviate eczema and even treat cold symptoms. It has powerful anti-cancer, anti-inflammatory, and immune-boosting properties. It's good for bone, teeth, skin, hair, and nails. Watercress can even help detoxify the liver.

The leaves of watercress are small and have a spicy or peppery taste.

Collard greens

In the United States, collard greens are most often used in Southern cooking, but they're gaining new respect as a nutritional powerhouse in any type of dish, including green smoothies. The large, thick leaves are loaded with disease-fighting beta carotene and vitamins A, C, E, and K. Collard greens are rich in zinc, magnesium, calcium, manganese, iron, phosphorus, and potassium. Add to that a high amount of fiber, natural immune-boosting properties, and powerful anti-inflammatory benefits, and you have a great green smoothie ingredient. Collard greens help reduce cell damage, hydrate skin, lower cholesterol, and can protect the body against arthritis, cardiovascular disease, cataracts, and macular degeneration.

Collard greens are large, flat, slightly bitter green leaves with a thick stem running down the middle. Look for the biggest, thickest leafy greens in your supermarket produce section; they're more than likely collard greens.

Celery

How many times have you thrown away celery leaves without realizing what a nutritious food they actually are? The leaves of celery are a great choice for green smoothies and a good way to prevent excess food from going to waste. The high levels of potassium and organic sodium in celery make it a great post-workout recovery food. Its powerful anti-inflammatory properties are particularly good in fighting bladder infections and urinary tract infections (UTIs), and reducing the pain and inflammation associated with arthritis and gout. Celery contains an active phytochemical called *coumarin,* which enhances the activity of cancer-fighting white blood cells. Celery is good against heartburn and indigestion, and it has even been touted as a natural aphrodisiac thanks to the *androsterone* (a potent male pheromone) it contains.

Look for celery stalks with plenty of leaves at your local farmers' market or in your local supermarket. Save the leaves on the stems for making smoothies.

Bok choy

Bok choy has been a staple food for health in China for more than 2,000 years, and it's still just as popular today. That probably has something to do with its wealth of vitamins A, C, and K; calcium; magnesium; potassium; manganese; and iron. Like broccoli and cauliflower, bok choy is a type of cabbage and a member of the cruciferous family of vegetables. Cruciferous vegetables are unique in that they're a rich source of sulfur-containing compounds known as *glucosinolates.* Glucosinolates have powerful anti-cancer benefits; they're especially effective against bladder cancer, breast cancer, colon cancer, and prostate cancer. Bok choy has a high concentration of antioxidants, anti-inflammatory benefits, and natural cholesterol-lowering abilities that help for cardiovascular support.

When eaten raw, bok choy tastes somewhat bitter. Overall, though, it's milder in taste than other greens.

Dandelion greens

Dandelions are often dismissed as an annoying weed, but fresh dandelion greens are actually an amazing health food packed with nutrients. They're exceptionally good for detoxifying the liver and have powerful anti-inflammatory and anti-cancer properties, especially for breast cancer and prostate cancer. Dandelion greens are a rich source of vitamins A and C, fiber, potassium, iron, calcium, magnesium, zinc, and phosphorus and have been used for centuries to treat anemia, scurvy, skin problems, blood disorders, digestive problems, and depression. They've even been shown to help regulate blood sugar and insulin levels.

The leaves have a mild, pleasant flavor, making them a great choice for green smoothies.

Only buy dandelion greens at farmers' markets, health food stores, or supermarkets. Picking your own can expose you to dangerous fertilizers.

Mustard greens

Mustard greens, a member of the cruciferous vegetable family, are best known for their anti-cancer effects. These benefits stem from mustard green's high amounts of disease-fighting antioxidants (including vitamins A, C, and E) and a naturally high level of glucosinolates. Mustard greens protect against breast cancer and heart disease and contain a high concentration of nutrients that are supportive for bone health — such as calcium, magnesium, and folate — so they're a good food choice for women going through menopause. They're also good for digestive health, healthy skin, and shiny, strong hair.

The leaves have a strong spicy flavor and combine best with sweet fruits such as mango, strawberries, pear, pineapple, or banana.

Turnip greens

No longer just a side dish, turnip greens are taking center stage as a disease-fighting, nutrient-dense food. (*Nutrient-dense* foods are those that contain a lot of nutrients in even a small serving.) One of the key features in turnip greens is the high calcium content, making these greens a great choice for strong bones and teeth. Their high amounts of vitamin A and lutein protect your eyes from macular degeneration. Turnip greens also give you omega-3 fatty acids to help reduce chronic oxidative stress (think of it as internal rust or damage to your cells) and chronic inflammation. The naturally high concentration of the antioxidant *kaempferol* in turnip greens can help lower women's risk of ovarian cancer.

As for the taste of turnip leaves, they're admittedly on the bitter and strong side. Try to mask the bitter flavor by combining the leaves with cinnamon, dates, peppermint oil, wild orange essential oil, or turmeric in your smoothie.

Beet greens

You probably already know that beets are good for your liver and overall health, but did you know that the real nutritional power is in the leafy greens? High in vitamins A, C, and K, beet greens are a powerhouse food that boosts the immune system and supports healthy skin, bones, teeth, and blood vessels. That makes them a good food for preventing osteoporosis, heart disease, high cholesterol, and cancer. Vitamin A is especially good if you have trouble with night vision, and vitamin K is an important element that aids in blood clotting. Beet greens also support liver detoxification and help relieve chronic constipation; their high iron content makes them beneficial for folks with anemia.

The taste of beet greens is on the bitter and somewhat earthy side. For that reason, combining the greens with sweeter fruits is your best bet. Strawberries, bananas, oranges, and raspberries work well with beet greens in smoothies.

But broccoli is green, too!

You may be wondering why some green foods, such as broccoli, Brussels sprouts, asparagus, peas, and green beans, didn't make the cut for green smoothies in this book. Although all green vegetables are excellent for health, not all of them digest well when paired with fruits. Leafy greens combine very well with fruits for digestion, but denser green veggies like broccoli or asparagus tend to ferment when combined with fruits. The result: excess gas and bloating. That's not a health concern, but it's still a not-so-pleasant memory of your first green smoothie experience. By all means, eat plenty of green veggies with other meals throughout the day, but to keep your stomach happy, use only leafy greens in your smoothies.

Alfalfa sprouts

Alfalfa sprouts are the shoots of the alfalfa plant, harvested before they become the full-grown plant. The sprouts are high in vitamins, minerals, essential fatty acids, protein, and fiber. In fact, alfalfa sprouts are the only plant that supplies the full range of vitamins, from vitamin A, C, E, and K to the B complex (even B12). Compounds called *saponins* in alfalfa sprouts have an antimicrobial and anti-inflammatory effect that helps reduce inflammation in the colon and supports the healing of ulcers, diverticulitis, and irritable bowel syndrome (IBS). Alfalfa sprouts are naturally high in *L-canavanine,* an amino acid beneficial in fighting leukemia, pancreatic and colon cancers, and certain types of breast tumors.

Their taste is slightly earthy, but you can easily mask it with fruits in a smoothie.

For some people, sprouts can be difficult to digest, resulting in excess gas or bloating. For that reason, I recommend you eat them in small amounts (½ cup or less) and combine them with natural digestive aids such as ginger, turmeric, or cinnamon in your smoothie.

Try adding other types of sprouts to your smoothie, including sunflower sprouts, radish sprouts, clover sprouts, broccoli sprouts, and even lentil or mung bean sprouts.

Fresh herbs

Using fresh herbs in a green smoothie is a great way to add more natural flavor, nutrients, and healing power. Here's a rundown of the best herbs for smoothies:

- ✔ **Parsley:** Parsley is high in vitamin C, is a natural cure for bad breath, helps reduce gas and aids in digestion, acts as a natural blood purifier, and is a good source of fiber. *Note:* Italian and flat-leaf parsley can be used interchangeably in green smoothie recipes.

- ✔ **Mint:** Mint is great for digestion, is a naturally alkalizing food, helps reduce allergy symptoms, aids in headache and pain relief, and contains natural anti-cancer benefits. (Flip to Chapter 1 for details on alkalinity.)

- ✔ **Basil:** Basil is an immune-boosting food, promotes cardiovascular health, and offers anti-inflammatory benefits that help with rheumatoid arthritis or inflammatory bowel conditions.

- ✔ **Fennel:** Fennel contains antiseptic and antiviral agents, is good for the immune system, promotes digestion, has natural anti-inflammatory benefits, and can help with menstrual disorders.

- ✔ **Oregano:** Oregano is high in antioxidants; acts as a natural antibacterial and antifungal agent; is a natural remedy against sore throat, asthma, colds, coughs, and flu; and provides a source of omega-3 fatty acids.

- ✔ **Cilantro:** Cilantro helps remove toxicity and heavy metals from your blood, is a natural digestive aid, has anti-inflammatory benefits, and helps regulate blood sugars.

- ✔ **Dill:** Dill helps relieve gas and indigestion; provides relief from menstrual disorders; prevents infection in the mouth, gums, and teeth; and has a calming effect good for sleep.

Lettuces

Adding lettuce to your green smoothie is another great option and helps bring variety to your leafy greens. When deciding which lettuce to use, look for darker, greener leaves for added minerals and chlorophyll. Iceberg lettuce, for example, isn't the best choice for smoothies because it's virtually all water and doesn't pack any punch of valuable nutrients. Plus, you're most likely eating iceberg lettuce already, and the whole point of having a green smoothie is to add more nutrients to your diet with greens that you don't normally eat. The following lettuces are good choices for smoothies:

- ✔ **Romaine:** Romaine lettuce is loaded with folate, vitamins C and K, antioxidants, and fiber; helps lower cholesterol and clean the digestive tract; and has a heart-healthy potassium content.

- ✔ **Arugula:** Arugula (also known as *rocket*) contains vitamins A, B, C, and K; is high in iron, calcium, phosphorous, potassium, magnesium, manganese, zinc, and copper; and is a powerful anti-cancer food.

✔ **Escarole:** Escarole is packed with antioxidants, helps clear acne, relieves constipation, cleanses the liver and gallbladder, is good for eye health, and has fantastic anti-cancer benefits.

Using Green Powders Rather than Fresh Greens

Nothing compares to the *bioavailability* of fresh leafy greens — that is, the rate at which your body can digest and absorb their nutrients. But realistically speaking, you may not always have access to fresh greens. Green powders can be a good alternative to fresh greens in winter months or while you're traveling; they're a practical way to still get some of the nutritional benefits of greens. You can also supplement a fresh-greens smoothie with a green powder, adding a dried green powder that you don't normally have in your diet as a way to increase variety in your greens. In that case, powdered greens such as spirulina, chlorella, wheatgrass, kelp, alfalfa, or barley grass are great choices. You can find out more about spirulina and chlorella powder in Chapter 6; I discuss wheatgrass powder in the next section.

Many green powders are sold as blends, with several greens mixed together. My favorite brands are from 100-percent certified organic companies like Navitas Naturals, HealthForce Nutritionals, and Amazing Grass. Whichever brands you choose, always try to buy products with the USDA 100 percent certified organic seal.

If you're a frequent traveler looking for an easy superfood green powder blend to take on the road, check out the individual green powder packets sold by Amazing Grass (http://amazinggrass. com/). Each packet is a single-size serving, so you can easily pack as many days as you need. Ask your hotel restaurant staff to make you a fresh fruit smoothie with water and your powder blend. You'll be surprised at how easy staying healthy on the road is!

Incorporating Wheatgrass

Wheatgrass is grown from the wheat seed (sometimes called *wheat berries*). Take the whole kernel of the wheat grain, soak it, sprout it, grow it in soil, and in just a few days, you've got fresh, emerald-green wheatgrass growing. Cut the grass at the base of the soil and put it in a juicer, and you're looking at one of the healthiest drinks on the planet. Fresh wheatgrass is always the best choice when it's available, but if you can't get fresh, choose powdered or frozen instead. The following sections explain the advantages of putting wheatgrass in your green smoothie and break down how to do so regardless of which form you use.

Eyeing wheatgrass's health benefits

Although it may look like regular backyard grass, wheatgrass is a different species of grass entirely; unlike your lawn grass, wheatgrass packs a real health punch. Wheatgrass juice nourishes your blood, cells, bones, hair, skin, teeth, kidneys, liver, and colon. It protects your lungs and blood from outside pollution, cigarette smoke, toxins, and heavy metals. Wheatgrass not only helps prevent disease but also helps reverse it.

More health benefits of wheatgrass juice include the following:

- It's a *complete protein,* meaning it contains all eight essential amino acids.
- It's packed with chlorophyll, a power anti-inflammatory agent and purifying element.
- It's mineral-rich; it contains more than 90 minerals your body needs.
- It's high in disease-fighting antioxidants that strengthen your immune system.
- It's full of beneficial enzymes that assist in different body functions, from healing after injuries to improving digestion and promoting weight loss.
- It helps rejuvenate aging cells and slow the aging process.
- It sweetens your breath and cleans your gums with natural antibacterial properties.
- It's naturally energizing without any caffeine.
- It promotes healthy intestinal flora (good bacteria in the gut).
- It's a powerful detoxifier for your liver and blood.
- It restores alkalinity to your blood and increases your red blood cell count.
- It strengthens the digestive tract and helps repair damage from ulcers and ulcerative colitis.

If you're gluten intolerant or suffer from celiac disease, avoid consuming any type of wheatgrass — fresh, dried, or frozen — or powder blends that contain wheatgrass powder. Technically speaking, wheatgrass doesn't contain any gluten. Gluten is found only in the wheat seed kernel (endosperm) and not in the stem or grass leaves. But there's no way to guarantee that no part of a seed is accidentally included in a wheatgrass product; the chance of cross-contamination is simply not worth the risk.

Never substitute wild or lawn grass for wheatgrass! Lawn grass isn't the same as wheatgrass and won't give you any health benefits. Harvesting unknown varieties of wild plants isn't safe. It exposes you to dangerous fertilizers and pesticides and puts you at a high risk of consuming an inedible or poisonous plant species.

Getting the most out of adding wheatgrass to a smoothie

The best way to consume wheatgrass is to cut it fresh and juice it immediately. That ensures you get the highest mineral, enzyme, antioxidant and vitamin concentration you can. Because the grass itself is so fibrous and, well, grasslike, you can't blend it up like you would other leafy greens. In fact, you can't even juice wheatgrass in a normal household (centrifugal) juicer; you'll likely end up ruining the motor if you try. Instead, you need either a specifically designed wheatgrass juicer or a masticating juicer that slow-presses to separate the liquid juice from the grassy fiber. My top recommendation for a slow-press masticating juicer is the Omega 8004. (Find more information on juicers and blenders in Chapter 2.)

If you're really keen to add fresh wheatgrass juice to your green smoothie, you can easily grow it yourself at home. If you don't have the time or resources to grow your own wheatgrass, you can buy freshly cut wheatgrass, take it home, and juice an ounce per day to add to your smoothie. Fresh-cut wheatgrass is sold near the fresh herbs and sprouts in the produce section of most health food stores and specialty supermarkets. (One pack of cut wheatgrass will typically make 4 to 6 ounces of fresh juice.)

If you don't have a masticating juicer, you have two other options. You can either buy frozen wheatgrass juice or use organic wheatgrass powder.

✓ **Frozen wheatgrass:** Look for frozen wheatgrass juice shots at your local health food store. In some cases, you may have to sign up to order a weekly tray. That means someone else grows it, cuts it, juices it, and freezes it, and all you need to do is add one frozen shot per smoothie.

✓ **Wheatgrass powder:** The easiest way to get wheatgrass in your smoothie is to use a 100 percent certified organic powder. Superfood companies such as Navitas Naturals, Amazing Grass, and HealthForce Nutritionals all sell top-quality wheatgrass powder. Add a teaspoon of wheatgrass powder to your smoothie per day. If the powder is a blend with other organic greens, add up to a tablespoon. Store wheatgrass powder in a cool place or refrigerate after opening.

Measuring out the right amount

Ben Franklin may not have been talking about wheatgrass when he said, "An ounce of prevention is worth a pound of cure," but he might as well have been. As I note in the preceding section, you only need to drink one ounce of fresh wheatgrass juice or one teaspoon of wheatgrass powder per day to reap its health rewards.

How much is one ounce? A typical shot glass varies between 1 and 1.5 ounces, so think of a shot of wheatgrass juice as a one-ounce serving.

Especially if you're new to wheatgrass, drinking an ounce of fresh juice per day is more than enough to start. If you try to drink too much wheatgrass at once, you can temporarily feel sick from the powerful and immediate detox effect, or cleansing reaction, that wheatgrass has on the liver (see the nearby sidebar on the Herxheimer effect). When it comes to drinking wheatgrass juice, less is definitely more. Over time, if you're feeling good, you can slowly increase to up to 2 to 3 ounces of fresh wheatgrass juice or 3 teaspoons of wheatgrass powder per day.

The Herxheimer effect: Experiencing a detox reaction

When your body gets a high dose of concentrated fresh chlorophyll, enzymes, and nutrients from raw leafy greens (especially fresh wheatgrass), you can sometimes experience a temporary detox or cleansing reaction as your body eliminates toxins, unwanted bacteria, microbes, and viruses. You may suffer from mild headaches, nausea, fatigue, dizziness, weakness, or even brain fog for a few hours or, in some cases, a few days. This temporary feeling of illness is known as the *Herxheimer effect* (named for 19th century doctor Karl Herxheimer), and it's actually an intense sign of healing. These reactions can indicate that your body has started to cleanse itself as it quickly tries to catch up on the overload of toxins being released.

If you experience any cleansing reactions, reduce your intake of greens by half to slow down the detox effect; you should also increase your water intake, practice lots of deep breathing, and get plenty of rest. After just a few days to a week, the cleansing reactions should pass. Before you know it, you'll feel increased energy and strength as a direct result of your body being cleaner inside!

Chapter 5

Deciding What to Use for Fruits and Sweeteners

In This Chapter

▶ Including fruits for added nutrition in smoothies

▶ Highlighting the health benefits of fruits

▶ Discovering other natural sweeteners

▶ Putting the kibosh on artificial sweeteners

*H*aving a green smoothie with just greens and water may be great for your health, but it can be a real challenge for your palate. Fruits offer a delicious and natural sweet taste that combines perfectly with the bitter taste of greens to give you a healthy and great-tasting smoothie. If your green smoothies taste good, you're much more likely to keep drinking them every day.

In addition to adding sweetness, fruits give you more fiber, more water, and a whole array of *phytochemicals* (natural, plant-based compounds) and disease-fighting micronutrients. The benefit to you: an even healthier health drink!

In this chapter, I highlight the most common fruits used in green smoothies and outline the health benefits of each. I explain why fruit is a beneficial ingredient in smoothies, and I try to dispel some of the myths surrounding fruit sugars and weight gain. The chapter also lists some alternative natural sweeteners that you can use in smoothies and explains why you should avoid using artificial sweeteners.

Boosting Smoothie Nutrition by Adding Fruits

You may think that most people would shy away from green smoothies because they're afraid of greens, but in my experience, the idea of adding fruit is what usually sends people running. How could that be? In a society both obsessed with diet and plagued by obesity, the thought of any type of sugar, even the healthy natural sugar in fruits, is immediately associated with weight gain. I've had countless students and clients tell me that they love the idea of having more greens in their diets, but they just can't put fruits in a smoothie for fear of gaining weight.

Before you lose yourself in the "no fruit" camp, consider a few facts:

✔ Combining the fructose in fruit with leafy greens and water gives you a high-fiber smoothie that's *not* overloaded with sugar.

✔ Fiber is the key component in fruit proven to regulate blood sugar levels and help with weight loss.

✔ The water in fruits helps keep you full, minimizing hunger (and perhaps unhealthy snacking) later in the day.

✔ The natural enzymes and alkalizing effects in fruit help you digest food better and faster. (Chapter 2 has more info on the benefits of alkaline pH.)

✔ Fruit contains many nutrients and antioxidants that offer invaluable health benefits.

✔ The sugars and lack of fiber in chocolate, coffee drinks, alcohol, cakes, cookies, cereals, and breads will make you gain weight faster than any fruit ever will!

When your body gets the nutrients it needs, you no longer feel hungry or think about food as much, and that alone can help you lose weight. With so much health to gain and potential weight to lose, fruits are actually the perfect addition to a green smoothie. And if certain fresh fruits aren't in season where you live, you can substitute frozen fruits (with no added sugar) for convenience.

Beyond an Apple a Day: Picking the Top Fruits for Your Smoothies

In this section, I highlight the most popular fruits to use in green smoothies. You really can't go wrong with any fruit you choose! Experimenting with different fruits is a great way to keep variety in your diet and to ensure that you're getting a wide spectrum of different vitamins, minerals, and antioxidants. So if you see a fruit listed here that you've never had before, search for it in your local supermarket and give it a try!

Banana

Bananas are undoubtedly one of the most popular fruits in the United States. In fact, on average, Americans eat more than 20 pounds of bananas per person per year, and it's easy to see why. The high amount of potassium in bananas makes them heart healthy and helps lower the risk of high blood pressure and stroke. Bananas are easy to digest and considered nonirritating for the stomach and upper gastrointestinal (GI) tract, so they're an excellent choice if you suffer from acid reflux, ulcers, colitis, or inflammation in the colon. Thanks to the combination of natural sugars, fiber, and potassium, bananas are great for sports endurance and recovery. Having a green smoothie made with bananas before or after your workout can give you more energy and improve your fitness performance.

The magnesium in bananas is a natural mood booster, helping alleviate symptoms of depression, anxiety, irritability, and other mood disorders. *Tryptophan* is an amino acid found in bananas that helps to increase serotonin levels, which in turn can reduce stress and regulate sleep patterns. Bananas are a good source of vitamin B6, important for creating hemoglobin for healthy blood. Vitamin C in bananas helps to boost the immune system and acts as a natural anti-inflammatory agent.

Apple

The old proverb about eating an apple a day dates back to the late 1800s and still applies today! Apples are cholesterol-free, sodium-free, and fat-free, and they're packed with vitamins A and C, antioxidants, and potassium. The fiber in apples helps cleanse and detoxify the colon, making them good for treating constipation, digestive disorders, and hemorrhoids. Pectin in apples offers cardiovascular benefits by reducing cholesterol levels.

High levels of boron in apples stimulate brain activity and increase mental alertness, making apples a real brain food. Boron also keeps your bones healthy and helps prevent osteoporosis by preserving calcium in the body. Apples have been shown to strengthen the heart, decrease mucous, help repair skin, and even lower the risk for respiratory diseases such as asthma. Eat your apples with the skin to get more nutrients; most of the antioxidants in apples are found in the skin.

Grapes

The ancient Greek gods symbolically ate grapes for love, fertility, and virility, and modern-day science can now prove that they made a wise choice. Grapes contain an antioxidant called *resveratrol* that offers vast health benefits. Resveratrol has been shown to boost egg quality and is good for male and female fertility by strengthening overall immune function. Recent studies show that resveratrol helps prevent certain types of cancer; it's particularly effective against breast cancer. It has also been shown to prevent the onset of Alzheimer's disease.

The antioxidants lutein and zeaxanthin in grapes are responsible for maintaining good eye health. Grapes are full of minerals such as copper, iron, and manganese, all of which are important for bone formation and strength. They're also rich in vitamins C, K, and A, making them one of the best foods for overall skincare. Red grapes contain antibacterial and antiviral properties, protecting you from infection and naturally boosting to the immune system. A well-known laxative, grapes are very effective in treating constipation. They're also good for relieving indigestion and irritation or inflammation of the stomach and digestive tract.

The darker a grape's color, the more phytonutrients it contains. Resveratrol is found in higher concentrations in red and purple grapes. The seeds of grapes (both red and green) also contain powerful antioxidant and immune-boosting properties. Get the biggest bang for your grape buck (or smoothie) by choosing red grapes with the seeds. Depending on what blender you use, the seeds may or may not fully blend, but they are edible and worth keeping in your smoothie for the added health benefits. If you can't get red grapes with the seeds, then seedless green grapes are still an excellent second choice.

Avocado

Adding fresh avocado to your lunchtime smoothie can help stabilize your blood sugar levels, minimize afternoon sugar cravings, and promote weight loss. Avocados contain *oleic acid,* a healthy fat that activates the part of your brain that makes you feel full. The fats in avocados are monounsaturated fats, or *good fats.* They promote heart health, lower blood pressure, and lower the risk for diabetes.

Avocados possess other great health benefits beyond healthy fat. In fact, many health experts refer to the avocado as the world's most perfect food! The high folate content in avocados makes them an excellent choice during pregnancy. Combine the folate with natural antioxidants such as lutein and glutathione and vitamin E, and you've got a fantastic, heart-healthy food that also protects against cataracts, macular degeneration, and certain types of cancer. Vitamin E is also known for its anti-aging properties, and the combination of vitamin E and omega-3 fatty acids in avocados has been found to reverse memory loss in Alzheimer's patients.

Pear

Hailed as "a gift of the gods" by the Greek poet Homer, pears have been considered a valuable health food since ancient times. Today, you can find more than 2,500 varieties of pears, so you definitely have a lot of options. Pears offer fantastic health benefits throughout every stage in life, from infancy to adulthood to a healthy old age. They're often recommended as a weaning food for babies because of their low acid content, ease of digestion, and minimal allergy risk. They cleanse the colon and act as a mild laxative, helping you maintain regularity and alleviating constipation. The fiber and antioxidants in pears help lower cholesterol and provide a boost to your immune system. Pears are rich in vitamins A, C, and E; niacin; folate; phosphorus; potassium; copper; calcium; iron; and magnesium. All these nutrients give pears substantial anti-inflammatory benefits that help treat chronic inflammation and prevent conditions such as asthma.

Pears also contain naturally high levels of boron (see the earlier section "Apple" for more on boron). The glutathione in pears assists in prevention of cardiovascular disease and stroke. In fact, the American Heart Association reports that eating fruits with white edible portions such as pears can reduce your risk of stroke by as much as 52 percent! The mild but sweet taste of pears makes them a perfect ingredient in green smoothies.

Lemon and lime

Both lemons and limes taste sour and acidic, but they're actually alkaline-forming because the stomach has to produce almost virtually no acid to digest them. Alkaline-forming foods are extremely valuable for maintaining a healthy pH, a strong immune system, good digestion, and effective absorption of nutrients. Lemons and limes are potent detoxifiers with a natural cleansing effect. They contain powerful antibacterial qualities that make them a natural purifier of the blood, liver, colon, and kidneys.

Lemons and limes are an excellent source of vitamin C, reducing inflammation and neutralizing free radical buildup in the body. The anti-inflammatory benefits are helpful for conditions such as osteoarthritis and rheumatoid arthritis. And the free-radical–fighting vitamin C, coupled with these fruits' outstanding phytonutrients, help combat cancer. The phytonutrients *limonoids* in particular have been shown to help fight cancers of the mouth, skin, lungs, blood, breast, stomach, and colon.

 If possible, use fresh lemons or limes in your smoothies and avoid using store-bought juice. Fresh-squeezed juice offers the highest amount of antioxidants, which means more healing power in your smoothie.

Orange

Oranges are among the most popular fruits worldwide because of their refreshingly sweet and satisfying taste. They also happen to be a powerhouse of nutrition, offering excellent anti-inflammatory and anti-cancer benefits and a reduced risk of cardiovascular disease. Like bananas (see the earlier section), oranges contain high amounts of heart-healthy potassium. Vitamin A in oranges helps maintain good vision, while vitamin C contributes to healthy, glowing skin. Oranges are also full of *beta carotene,* a powerful antioxidant that encourages eye health, protects the cells and skin from free radical damage, and prevents signs of aging. Oranges are similar to lemons and limes in that they're one of the most alkaline-forming foods available.

Either you can squeeze fresh orange juice into your smoothie or peel the skin, remove the seeds, and add the whole orange. A high-powered blender will have no problem pulverizing an orange with the pith (the white outer skin), but a standard household blender may leave some larger, chunky bits from the pith in your smoothie. If you have a standard household blender and want to blend a whole orange, I recommend you add another ½ cup of water to the recipe. Otherwise, just use the juice.

Kiwi

Despite the name, kiwis aren't native to New Zealand. In fact, the seeds were originally imported from China, and the fruit was previously called the Chinese gooseberry. Although small in size, the kiwi offers a huge array of health benefits. Kiwis are an excellent source of vitamin C, and actually, ounce for ounce, they contain more vitamin C than oranges. Kiwis also contain high amounts of antioxidants, helping to maintain eye health and a strong immune system. The potassium in kiwis makes them great for protecting cardiovascular health and keeping cholesterol levels in check. The taste is really delicious in a green smoothie as it brings a combination of sweet with an almost creamy texture when blended. To ensure a clean fruit that's free of chemical residue, peel the outer brown skin with a knife and use only the inner green fruit in your smoothies.

Grapefruit

This large fruit tastes just like paradise, as its Latin name *Citrus paradisi* suggests. Grapefruit has long been known to promote weight loss, mainly because it's low in sodium, high in fat-burning enzymes, and low on the glycemic index (GI). (The *glycemic index* is a way of measuring how foods that contain carbohydrates affect your blood sugar; lower values are better.) The low GI, high fiber, and high water content in grapefruit make it an excellent fruit choice for diabetics. (Refer to Chapter 13 for some smoothie recipes for diabetics.) Even more good news for diabetics: *Naringenin,* the antioxidant that gives grapefruit a naturally bitter taste, has been found to improve insulin sensitivity and glucose tolerance. Like oranges, grapefruit's beta carotene promotes eye health.

Grapefruit contains limonoids and pectin, both of which support cardiovascular health and have powerful anti-cancer benefits. They're also packed with vitamin C, which supports a healthy immune system and lowers your risk of heart disease, cancer, and stroke. The combination of vitamin C and other powerful antioxidants in grapefruit stimulates natural cleansing and liver detoxification. The vitamin C in grapefruit has also been linked to a reduced risk of developing kidney stones. *Lycopene,* a pigment that gives grapefruit its red color, is known as a powerful agent against inflammation, tumors, and cancer.

Berries

What berries may lack in size, they certainly make up for in nutrients. The star nutrient in berries is *anthocyanins,* powerful antioxidant and anti-inflammatory chemicals that give berries their bright red, blue, and purple colors. Anthocyanins provide a vast spectrum of healing support, from bone health and cardiovascular benefits to protection from macular degeneration and decreased risk of cancer. Berries are considered low in terms of their glycemic index, giving them a favorable impact on blood sugar regulation and making them a naturally good choice for diabetics.

Here are some of the most commonly used berries in green smoothies. Other smoothie-friendly berries include huckleberries, cranberries, bilberries, mulberries, and currants.

- ✔ **Strawberries:** Strawberries are an excellent source of vitamin C, helping to protect the eyes and skin from free radical damage, boosting the immune system, and offering natural anti-inflammatory benefits. They're also a good source of folate, which helps in treating atherosclerosis and rheumatoid arthritis. Potassium in strawberries helps to minimize bone loss and offers cardiovascular benefits.

- ✔ **Blueberries:** Blueberries are truly little blue bundles of health, packed with manganese, vitamin K, and antioxidants. Research suggests that a blueberry-rich diet improves motor skills and helps fight diseases such as cancer, heart disease, and diabetes. They're good for your skin, and they boost your brain.

✔ **Raspberries:** Raspberries offer an ample supply of manganese, a mineral that helps to decrease premenstrual syndrome symptoms, improve bone health, and decrease pain associated with arthritis. Raspberries are high in vitamin C and *ellagic acid,* a type of antioxidant that has powerful anti-carcinogenic, antibacterial, and antiviral properties. Red raspberries are the most commercially available variety of raspberry. Black raspberries are smaller in size than red raspberries but are packed with even higher amounts of ellagic acid.

✔ **Blackberries:** Studies show blackberries have one of the highest antioxidant contents per serving of any food. Like raspberries, they're also high in ellagic acid. Blackberries tend to be larger in size than raspberries. The taste varies from bitter to sweet depending on how ripe they are when picked.

Peach and nectarine

The major difference between nectarines and peaches is that nectarines have smooth skins, while the skin of peaches is soft and fuzzy. Both are *stone fruits,* meaning they have a large stone seed in their inner core. Summertime is the season for stone fruits, so that's a great time to start adding them to your smoothies.

Both peaches and nectarines are good sources of fiber and vitamins A and C. The enzymes and fiber in peaches and nectarines assist in maintaining healthy bowel function and relieving constipation. Their high potassium content plays an important role in maintaining good muscle, heart, and kidney health. Peaches and nectarines are a good source of beta carotene. Both fruits are also great for the skin.

Plum

Plums are another type of stone fruit, one with a naturally sweet and tart taste. They're a good source of fiber; potassium; iron; and vitamins A, C, and K. High in antioxidants, plums are excellent for eyesight; clear skin; strong, thick hair; good bone density; heart health; regular bowel function; and improved blood circulation. Plums are a good choice for diabetics because they're low on the glycemic index and can help control blood sugar levels. Some studies have connected plums to cancer prevention, especially for breast, lung, and gastrointestinal cancers.

Don't peel your plums; most of the powerful antioxidants are in the skin. Prunes are the dried version of plums and can also be used in smoothies. Substitute three whole dried prunes for two fresh plums in recipes.

Apricot

Apricots may be small, but you shouldn't overlook their health benefits. These stone fruits are naturally high in iron, making them a good source of plant-based iron for vegans and vegetarians. They're rich in fiber; antioxidants; and vitamins A, C, and E. Apricots promote eye health, skin health, bone health, and heart health and help protect against cancer.

Dried apricots are a suitable substitute for fresh apricots as long as they're organic. Non-organic dried apricots contain high levels of sulfur dioxide as a preservative and can cause adverse reactions, especially if you suffer from asthma or allergies. Substitute two organic dried apricots for one fresh apricot in recipes.

Papaya

Christopher Columbus once called papaya the "fruit of the angels" after seeing native islanders thrive on it. This tropical, nutrient-packed fruit contains several enzymes — most notably *papain,* a proteolytic enzyme that helps break down the food you eat. (*Proteolytic enzymes* destroy the defense shields of viruses, tumors, allergens, yeasts, and various forms of fungus.) Papain has been shown to reduce acid reflux and indigestion and can even relieve ulcers and irritable bowel syndrome. Combine that with the high amounts of antioxidants in papaya, and you have a fantastic anti-cancer food.

Papaya also has powerful anti-inflammatory benefits, making it good for many other ailments, including atherosclerosis, heart disease, and rheumatoid arthritis. The fruit is high in vitamins C, A, and E; folate; fiber; and potassium, all of which contribute to clear skin, good eyesight, healthy hair, and a strong immune system.

Save overripe fruits and avoid mushiness

Fresh fruit is always best (because of its enzymes and its easier digestibility), but don't let your overripe fruits go to waste! When your fruit starts getting soft, cut it into pieces and put them in a zip-top bag in the freezer. That's the fruit you can use in a green smoothie later, on a day when you don't have any fresh fruit at home or when you want a colder, frozen smoothie. Some people even bag various fruits together so they can grab one bag when they want a fast and easy green smoothie later.

Only freeze the parts you want to add to your smoothie. Always peel bananas and remove any cores, seeds, or stones in other fruits. Cut away any bruised or brown bits of the flesh.

The small, black seeds in papaya taste quite peppery and contain powerful antibacterial effects. Try adding just two to three papaya seeds to your smoothie for an extra detoxifying boost.

Pineapple

Pineapple is one of the most popular tropical fruits in the world. It contains *bromelain,* a proteolytic enzyme that works to improve digestion and maintain healthy bowel function. (The preceding section has more on this type of enzyme.) The manganese and vitamins C and A in pineapple help fight colds and flus, strengthen bones, decrease your risk of macular degeneration, alleviate arthritis, prevent infection, and strengthen immune function.

Mango

Mangoes are a delightful tropical fruit, rich in aromatic flavor and full of health benefits. Mangoes contain *gallic acid,* a type of antioxidant with antifungal and antiviral properties that's also good for the digestive tract. They also contain tartaric acid, malic acid, and citric acid that help your body maintain a natural alkaline reserve. (Check out Chapter 1 for more on alkaline pH.) Vitamin A and beta carotene in mangoes help in rejuvenating and moisturizing your skin. Vitamin B6 in mangoes improves brain function, elevates mood, and controls stress. And eating mangoes protects your body against the risk of certain types of cancer — including colon cancer, breast cancer, leukemia, and prostate cancer — because of the fruit's antioxidants.

Cantaloupe

Cantaloupe, sometimes called *muskmelon,* is packed with high amounts of vitamin A, a powerful antioxidant for improving eye health. The antioxidants in cantaloupe also help protect your cells from free radical damage and oxidative stress, giving the fruit potent anti-aging and anti-cancer benefits. That's why cantaloupe is a top choice to help prevent wrinkles and skin cancer. Vitamin C in cantaloupes supports a strong immune system, and the potassium is good for cardiovascular health.

This deliciously sweet fruit has been shown to improve lung health for smokers and can help those quitting smoking recover from nicotine withdrawal by replenishing their supply of vitamin A and beta carotene. The high fiber, enzymes, and water content in cantaloupe can reduce feelings of hunger and are essential for good digestive health. Cantaloupe also contains a lipid known as *myo-inositol* that may aid in reducing symptoms of anxiety and insomnia.

Honeydew is another type of muskmelon closely related to the cantaloupe. Besides the difference in color (honeydew is light green inside whereas cantaloupe is a more pale orange), the melons offer nearly identical health benefits. The taste of honeydew is a bit sweeter because it usually contains slightly more natural sugar than cantaloupe. Either melon is a good choice depending on what's fresh and available in your local area.

Did you know that cantaloupe is actually a member of the cucumber family? For details on its slender green cousin, head to the later section "Cucumber."

Watermelon

You may think of watermelon as a fantastic summer treat, but it offers much more than just a refreshing snack on a hot day. The red color in watermelon comes from its high levels of lycopene, an important nutrient for cardiovascular health and particularly beneficial in reducing inflammation and neutralizing free radicals. Watermelon also contains *L-citrulline,* an amino acid shown to reduce the accumulation of fat in fat cells. L-citrulline has also been found to help your body remove lactic acid more quickly, which means a faster recovery time and less muscle soreness after a tough workout.

Watermelon is a natural detoxifier for the liver and kidney because it helps the body flush out excess acid waste. It's also high in vitamins A, C, and B6; potassium; calcium; and beta carotene, making watermelon a good choice for bone health, healthy skin and hair, improved eyesight, and immune support.

Mixing melons with other fruits

The high enzyme and water content in melons makes them digest quickly through the colon, and that's a good thing! But combining them with other foods can slow down their ability to break down, causing fermentation in your gut and perhaps leading to excess gas or bloating. The highest chance of fermentation happens when you combine sugars (such as those in melons) with fats (such as milk, yogurt, or even avocado). So when putting melon in your smoothie, focus on using lowfat ingredients. (Leafy greens are the universal combiner. They combine well with everything, so you don't have to worry about the effects of mixing them with melon.)

Pomegranate

Some studies suggest that pomegranate juice contains almost three times as many antioxidants as green tea or red wine. The fruit's small red seeds are loaded with disease-fighting antioxidants and flavonoids that offer protection against cardiovascular disease, osteoarthritis, diabetes, and several different types of cancer. In particular, pomegranate contains *punicalagins,* unique antioxidants that have antifungal and antibacterial properties. Studies have shown pomegranate to be effective in fighting the return of prostate cancer among men who have had surgery or radiation for the disease.

If you're looking to reduce wrinkles, increase production of collagen, heal scarring on the skin, clear skin blemishes, or slow the process of skin aging, then pomegranate is the fruit for you.

The seeds of the pomegranate are the part you want to add to a smoothie. To remove them, cut the fruit in half, break the sections apart, and submerge each half in a bowl of water to contain any juice spatter as you gently pry the seeds out using your fingers. The seeds will float in the water for easy collection.

Persimmon

Look for an orange fruit that resembles a tomato, and you've got persimmon, a delicious fruit loaded with antioxidants, vitamins A and C, phosphorous, manganese, potassium, copper, and fiber. When ripe, the flavor of persimmon is somewhat like a dense, sweet cinnamon apple. Persimmon is used as a traditional remedy for treating constipation, diarrhea, and hemorrhoids. It's also been shown effective for lung infections and asthma. In China, persimmon is combined with fresh ginger in tea as a natural remedy for hiccups.

The high vitamin A content, combined with antioxidants, gives the persimmon its anti-cancer properties. One study showed that the skin of the persimmon contains potent phytochemicals to protect cells against oxidative stress and damage associated with aging.

Depending on the variety of persimmons you buy, they may or may not contain large seeds. To add persimmon to your smoothie, cut the fruit into quarters, discarding the stem and removing any seeds.

Cucumber

Yes, that's right . . . cucumber is actually a fruit! How does that work? The general rule is that if the edible part of a plant has seeds, the plant is classified as a fruit. If the edible part is seedless, the plant is a vegetable. (Genetically modifying a fruit to have no seeds doesn't count.)

Cucumbers are 95 percent water, keeping the body and skin hydrated, flushing out toxins, and in some cases, even helping to dissolve kidney stones. Because of their low calorie and high water content, cucumbers are an ideal choice for people trying to lose weight. They contain ample amounts of potassium, magnesium, and fiber, working effectively to regulate blood pressure. The high silicon content helps relieve joint pain, strengthen connective tissue, and can be good for treating arthritis. Cucumbers have no sugar, so they're a great food for controlling blood sugar. They also contain a hormone that supports the pancreas with insulin production.

 If you tend to get gas or indigestion from eating cucumbers, it's most likely from the skin. Cucumbers contain *cucurbitacin,* a substance that causes burping and indigestion and also contributes to that bitter taste cucumbers sometimes have. Most of the cucurbitacin is in the peel, outer flesh, and stem ends of cucumbers. So if you want to avoid stomach pains but still eat cucumbers, you should peel the skin.

Tomato

Tomato is a savory fruit with an array of health benefits. Lycopene is the powerful antioxidant that gives tomatoes a bright red color. Studies have shown that a diet rich in lycopene-containing foods can help reduce the risk of prostate, breast, lung, colon, and pancreatic cancer. Lycopene also helps lower cholesterol, reduce inflammation, improve immune function, and prevent blood from clotting. Other disease-fighting nutrients found in tomatoes include vitamins A, B6, and C; beta carotene; potassium; niacin; and folate.

Bell pepper

Bell peppers are also in the fruit family and are most commonly in found in green, red, orange, or yellow colors. Full of vitamins and antioxidants, bell peppers promote heart health, contain anti-inflammatory and anti-cancer benefits, help to protect the skin and eyes, and are a good choice for diabetics and weight loss. Red bell peppers are sweeter and offer the most nutritional benefits, while the more bitter-tasting green pepper offers the least.

Not all green smoothies are green

As you start making green smoothies, you may notice that sometimes your smoothie isn't actually green in color. Depending on what fruit and superfoods you use, you can have green smoothies that are yellowish-green and even purple. Fresh berries such as blueberries, raspberries, strawberries, or blackberries tend to give smoothies a more reddish-brown color in spite of the fresh greens you add. Don't let the color fool you! If you added fresh greens, it's still a green smoothie.

Considering Other Natural Sweetening Options

Using fresh fruits such banana, apple, pineapple, or mango in a green smoothie makes a naturally sweet, delicious health drink that you really don't need to add extra sweeteners (or additional calories) to. Especially if you're trying to lose or maintain your weight, be cautious of adding more sweetening agents to your smoothies. However, if you're using bitter greens such as watercress or collard greens and want to hide the bitterness with an added dash of sweetness, try focusing on natural sweeteners such as the ones listed in this section.

Avoid using refined table sugar, an ingredient that contains empty calories, promotes weight gain, disrupts insulin levels, is addictive, and can increase cholesterol levels.

Raw honey

Honey is nature's miracle food; it's known for its natural antiseptic, anti-inflammatory, and antibacterial properties and has been used as a health food worldwide for more than 4,000 years. When taken orally, honey can be used to treat stomach ulcers, sore throat, strep throat, acid reflux, and gastrointestinal disorders. It's also an effective cough suppressant and can help alleviate symptoms of seasonal allergies.

Raw honey is the unpasteurized version of the more commonly used heat-treated and refined honey you see at the store. Raw honey has gone through added filtration, which mainly helps extend shelf life but also gives it more antioxidants and health benefits than normal honey. *Manuka honey* is a unique variety of raw honey manufactured in New Zealand; it has exceptional healing power because of a very high concentration of *methylglyoxal* (MGO), the compound that gives honey its antibacterial properties.

Add 2 tablespoons of raw honey to your smoothie for a sweeter drink and lots of side bonus health benefits, too.

If you're allergic to bees or suspect that you're allergic to bees, don't consume honey or any bee products.

Stevia

Stevia is the best natural sweetener if you have diabetes, high cholesterol, or are trying to lose weight. *Stevia* is a plant native to South America with leaves that contain a naturally sweet compound called *steviol glycosides.* In fact, stevia leaves are so sweet that they're 30 to 50 times sweeter than sucrose (table sugar)! Unlike synthetic sweeteners, stevia has no side effects. Even better, stevia has a glycemic index of 0 and is a low-calorie, noncarcinogenic sweetening option that helps stabilize blood sugar levels, reduce blood pressure, and treat heartburn and indigestion.

Find stevia in green leaf, liquid extract, or powder form in the sweetener section of health food stores or larger supermarkets. Of all forms, the most commonly used is powdered stevia. Adding just a teaspoon of stevia powder gives you a burst of sweet flavor in your green smoothie.

Dates

Dates are a fantastically sweet desert fruit sold in dried form, and Medjool dates are the most common variety available. Dates are high in fiber, potassium, copper, manganese, and magnesium and are especially known for promoting healthy bowel function. The high natural sulfur in dates helps reduce seasonal allergies. The high sugar in dates makes them perfect for an immediate energy boost.

Dates can also promote weight gain if you aren't careful. If you're watching your waistline, limit your intake to only one date per day. Otherwise, you can add two to three dates to your smoothie.

Agave nectar

I include agave nectar in this section because many people mistakenly think that it's a healthy option for a natural sweetener, but recent studies now show that it's not. In fact, almost all commercially available agave nectar is processed in the same way as high fructose corn syrup (HCFS), giving agave nectar the highest fructose content of any commercially available sweetener (with the exception of pure liquid fructose).

Agave nectar is made from made from the starchy root of the *agave* plant, a type of cactus native to Mexico. Although agave nectar is marketed as a low glycemic index food suitable for diabetics, the high fructose content definitely makes its health benefits questionable. If you choose to eat it, use it sparingly — not more than one to two tablespoons in a smoothie per day.

Avoiding Artificial Sweeteners

Although artificial sweeteners such as aspartame, saccharin, sorbitol, neotame, and sucralose are approved by the FDA and considered safe for human consumption, growing evidence suggests that many of these laboratory-created products may be harmful to your health. Studies have proven that several of these sweeteners are actually carcinogenic and can cause damage to the kidneys. Some artificial sweeteners have been shown to trigger mood changes, panic attacks, dizziness, nervousness, memory impairment, nausea, depression, seizures, numbness, rashes, insomnia, hearing loss, vertigo, and loss of taste. Other studies show that artificial sweeteners can trigger more sugar and carbohydrate cravings after eating them.

I don't know about you, but to me it just doesn't seem worth the risk to start adding these to your diet, especially when fresh, all natural fruits have so many naturally sweet flavors that don't have any harmful side effects. If you're looking to reduce calories, sweeten your smoothies with low-sugar ingredients such as blueberries, grapefruit, cucumber, tomato, or bell pepper. Choosing all-natural options gives you the highest chances of keeping your most valuable asset — your health — for many years to come.

Chapter 6

Adding Superfoods, Medicinal Ingredients, Liquids, and More

*O*ne of the best parts about drinking a green smoothie is that you can add extras to your smoothie to make it even more nutritious and to suit your individual dietary needs. By adding superfoods and other supplements, you can turn your green smoothie into a one-stop shop for getting at least your minimum daily requirements of minerals and vitamins. If you drink such a smoothie every day, you're setting yourself up long-term to have a stronger immune system, better digestion, and increased energy. And that's definitely a good thing!

If you've already been reading about powders, proteins, and health drinks, you know that everything these days seems to be marketed as a superfood. Even coffee has been called a superfood, but that's not something you'd add to a green smoothies — or is it? This chapter explains what superfoods can do for you, whether you even need them, and which ones you can start adding to your daily green smoothie. I outline the most popular superfoods from various cultures around the world and what superfoods you can find in your local farmers' market just down the road. I also weigh in on whether supplements are appropriate for green smoothies and help you make smarter choices when you're trying to sift through what's available.

With all this excitement over green smoothies, you may be tempted to start throwing everything in the blender with the idea that more is more. Well, that's not always the case, so here, I clarify why keeping certain items out of your green smoothie is a good idea. With just the right balance of good ingredients, you're sure to stay on track and get the results you desire. Here's to your health!

Looking at the Pros and Cons of Eating Superfoods

A *superfood* is a natural food with exceptionally high concentrations of vitamins, minerals, antioxidants, trace minerals, enzymes, proteins, or special healing benefits. Regular food becomes a superfood when it's *nutritionally dense* for its particular size and weight. That means that compared to other foods of the same size, a superfood contains even more nutrition and healing power. Think of the difference between regular fuel and premium fuel for your car. That's the same logic applied to normal food versus superfoods.

Different cultures around the world have cultivated their own superfoods for centuries; the traditions of eating these foods when sick or diseased have been passed from generation to generation. They've become a natural part of the local diet as well. On a daily basis, people eat a small amount of their local superfood for preventative maintenance as a natural way to stay healthy and strong. Goji berries, for example, are used in traditional Chinese medicine to help eyesight, boost immune function, improve circulation, and promote longevity. Maca root is known in the Incan and Peruvian culture as the "Peruvian ginseng," a powerful healing food said to increase stamina and energy, improve libido, enhance fertility, and promote anti-aging. In the Hunza Valley of Pakistan, where people live to be well older than 100 years old and cancer is nearly nonexistent, freshly ground flaxseed is a staple in the daily diet.

The popularity of superfoods has skyrocketed because of a combination of the growing interest in natural foods and healing methods and the modern-day ease of exporting and transporting foods from all over the world. Everyone can enjoy more of the world's healthiest foods in his or her diet simply because getting them is now fast and easy. The following sections explore the arguments for and against eating superfoods and touch on how to easily coordinate them into green smoothies.

Making a case for adding superfoods to your diet

Superfoods are especially good for anyone trying to reclaim health, increase energy levels, improve endurance, prevent disease, or simply feel better. More nutrition means better health and well-being. It's that easy.

However, some people argue that eating foods from all over the world isn't natural. For example, they say that eating goji berries from China when you live all the way across the world in Colorado doesn't make sense because you're not only increasing your over-all carbon footprint but also eating a food that is neither local nor freshly available in your region. (For more on carbon footprints, see the sidebar "What is a carbon footprint?")

I advocate eating local and fresh wherever possible, especially for fruits, vegetables, and greens. Eating more local foods helps your immune system adjust to seasonal pollens and decreases your risk of allergies. But fresh, local foods often aren't enough to keep people healthy; most people simply don't have time to prepare a lot of fresh food at home, and in most countries around the globe, fresh food doesn't even grow in winter months.

And consider another factor I've seen time and time again while preparing nutrition plans for thousands of clients from all over the globe: In today's modern, busy world, most people are deficient in minerals and vitamins — a situation worsened by the stressed-out lifestyles so many people live. Life doesn't look like it's going to slow down anytime soon, so taking a practical approach to nutrition is important. That's where superfoods really can help you live a better, longer, healthier life.

What is a carbon footprint?

The term *carbon footprint* refers to the amount of greenhouse gases (specifically carbon dioxide) emitted by a person's activities or a product's manufacture and transport during a certain period of time.

Consider this example: Food grown in China has to be driven to a port, placed on a ship, transported across the globe, distributed by truck to a supermarket ware-house, and eventually delivered to a local store. If you add up all the emissions released from the first truck, the ship, the second truck, and the third truck to get that food from its origin to your supermarket, you can see that it has a much higher carbon footprint than a food that was grown on a local farm and delivered by only one truck to your local farmers' market.

Not all superfoods are recommended for pregnant and/or breastfeeding women. Check out Chapter 15 for more specific advice on green smoothies and foods for fertility, pregnancy, and breastfeeding.

Balancing superfoods with the rest of your diet

Everyone can benefit from superfoods, but you shouldn't eat a diet of *only* superfoods. Fresh fruits, vegetables, nuts, seeds, and grains provide the foundation of a balanced diet for good health. Look at superfoods as a way to add to that healthy foundation and take your health to a whole new level.

Many superfoods are sold in powder form to preserve their freshness and make them easy to ship across the world. Having a diet of *only* powders isn't good for your body long term because you need natural, whole fiber in your diet, and you need to use your teeth to chew food, too!

As for how many superfoods to consume, try to be practical in your approach. Adding too many superfoods to your diet makes you much more likely to crash and burn because you grow tired of having to remember all the different powders and extra foods to take every day! But you're not likely to experience any noticeable health benefits if you have only one superfood per day. However, if your budget only allows you to start with one or two superfoods, taking what you can is perfectly fine. Even adding a small amount of extra antioxidants, vitamins, minerals, and healing power can definitely make a difference.

If you're ready to take the jump, focus on trying three to four superfoods per day. With that amount, you're getting a high boost of nutrition, you're choosing a manageable number of new foods to add to your diet, and you're creating a new healthy habit that you can easily maintain for life. Because superfoods are so nutritionally dense, you don't have to eat a large quantity or serving to reap the health benefits. Follow the recommended dosage suggested on each individual product.

Keep your superfoods fresher longer by transferring them to glass containers or jars and storing them in the refrigerator or freezer. Glass containers are the safest choice for storing foods because unlike certain plastics, glass can't leach chemicals into the food. Save money on containers by recycling your own jars; clean them thoroughly and use them to store your new superfoods at home.

Examining Top Superfoods for Green Smoothies

If you use a balanced healthy diet as a base and add superfoods to get even more nutrients, you can really start to feel a difference. Trying to use superfoods to make up for an unhealthy diet full of fried, processed, or nutrient-deficient foods doesn't offer any long-term positive results. To get the best results, use superfoods as a way to *complement* your current healthy diet.

Superfoods are great to add to your diet if you can't afford to eat 100-percent organic foods. Adding some extra support on a daily basis means you're still getting that high-boost of nutrients your body needs.

Here are some great superfoods you can easily add to your green smoothie for a daily dose of natural nutrition. **Remember:** You don't have to add all these superfoods to your green smoothie every day. Try to find three to four superfoods that will help you achieve your individual health goals and start there. To maintain variety in your diet and to keep things interesting, you can switch out for a new or different superfood each time you're ready to buy more.

Spirulina

Spirulina is a blue-green algae that grows in fresh water. It's a complete vegetable protein and a source of practically all the vitamins, minerals, digestive enzymes, and trace elements your body needs. Spirulina is especially high in iron, magnesium, manganese, zinc, and potassium. The chlorophyll in spirulina naturally cleanses the blood and detoxifies the body.

Spirulina is cultivated, dried, and sold in powder, tablet, capsule, and even crunchy forms. You can find it at your local health food store. The easiest way to use it in a smoothie is to add a teaspoon of spirulina powder to the ingredients.

The taste of spirulina can initially be, well, a bit disgusting. Many people say that it smells and tastes like "pond scum" or "dirty fish tank." Don't be discouraged by the taste! You can actually hide the strong taste of spirulina in your smoothie by blending it with sweet fruits such as pineapple, mango, orange, or banana. Higher-quality spirulina (either grown in Hawaii or grown organically) tends to have a better, less fishy taste than the cheaper, generic brands.

Chlorella

Chlorella is a green algae that grows in fresh water. It has the highest concentrations of chlorophyll of any plant in the world; it's also very high in magnesium and is a good source of plant-based protein. Chlorella is good for digestive support because it stimulates the growth of good gut bacteria in the digestive system.

Consuming chlorophyll can increase your energy levels; aid in digestion; support immune function; and help in fighting major lifestyle diseases such as Type-2 diabetes, cardiovascular disease, and obesity.

Chlorella generally comes in tablet form, but you can also occasionally find it as a loose powder. You can buy it online or at your local health food store. Add a teaspoon of chlorella powder or three to four chlorella tablets to your smoothie.

Aloe vera

Aloe vera has amazing anti-inflammatory, antibacterial, and antifungal properties. Fresh aloe vera helps digestion and elimination; boosts the immune system; and is highly effective at healing, moisturizing, and rejuvenating the skin.

Aloe vera is best when eaten fresh, and some supermarkets and health food stores sell fresh aloe vera leaves. You can also grow your own aloe vera at home; just be sure to avoid using any chemical fertilizers. When preparing fresh aloe vera to add to a green smoothie, peel away the green outer skin of a 1-inch-x-1-inch piece and use only the inner gel.

The other alternative is to buy aloe vera juice concentrate and dilute it in your smoothie. (You can also dilute the concentrate with water or juice to drink if you're not making a green smoothie.) Aloe vera juice is available at most local health food stores.

 Aloe vera is quite strong and can cause stomach cramps if taken in large amounts. Always start with a teaspoon of either fresh aloe vera or aloe juice concentrate daily and gradually increase the amount you consume, up to two tablespoons per day.

 Use only fresh aloe vera or aloe vera juice in your green smoothie. Don't use any aloe gels or after-sun aloe creams. Those products aren't safe for human consumption because they contain alcohol, preservatives, perfumes, and other chemicals. You can safely apply aloe gel or cream to your skin, but don't ingest it.

Free radicals versus antioxidants

Free radicals develop because of internal oxidation from the buildup of toxins such as drugs, alcohol, and chemicals in body products and food. Stress, poor air quality, and frequent travel on planes can all increase the formation of free radicals in the body. It's like your car getting rustier and rustier over time, except this "rust" is happening on the inside of your body. Eventually, these free radicals can impair your immune system and make it more difficult for the body to fight disease.

Antioxidants are substances found in natural, whole foods, and they help break down free-radical damage in the body. Adding high antioxidant superfoods to your diet can help strengthen your immune system, decrease signs of aging, prevent disease, and even improve liver function. It's a small investment to make with a high return: your health!

Acai powder

Acai (pronounced ah-sigh-*ee*) is an Amazonian berry native to South America; it contains the richest source of anthocyanins in any food. *Anthocyanins* are the powerful antioxidants found in red wine (they're what make red wine red and are also found in other foods such as purple cabbage, eggplants, and blueberries). The powerful antioxidants in acai berries naturally fight off aging, inflammation, and cancer. The berries are also a source of calcium, vitamin E, and phosphorous.

Adding acai to your diet is a good idea as preventative maintenance during flu season, during times of stress, or just before and after travel. People recovering from illness or surgery can take acai powder to help the body heal and to strengthen their overall immune systems.

Acai powder is available in any health food store and is typically sold in powder form. Add two to three teaspoons to your smoothie.

Bee pollen

Bee pollen is a magical combination of flower pollen collected by bees and mixed with nectar and bee enzymes. It contains high amounts of minerals, vitamins, and enzymes. Because of its exceptionally high nutrient content, bee pollen is often referred to as "nature's most complete food."

The health benefits of bee pollen include increasing energy levels and endurance, balancing metabolism, strengthening your immune system, repairing skin damage, improving fertility and prostate function, building natural resistance to allergies (particularly hay fever), and reducing symptoms of asthma.

Anyone with an allergy to bees or pollen should avoid eating any bee pollen. If you've never had bee pollen before, be sure to take a tolerance test to determine whether you have any allergic reaction. Place one or two grains of pollen on your tongue and wait a few minutes. If nothing happens, chew them up and wait again. If you experience any watery eyes; sneezing; or swelling of the mouth, lips, or tongue, then you have a potential allergy to pollen.

You can find bee pollen in health food stores, farmers' markets, and some grocery stores. It's most commonly sold in granule form but also comes in powder form. Always start with small amounts of bee pollen (less than a half teaspoon) and gradually build up to taking more, up to two tablespoons daily.

Flaxseed

Flaxseed (or *linseed*) is a very small, shiny seed with a lot of great health benefits, from reducing cholesterol to improving blood sugar levels for diabetics. Flax is very high in dietary fiber, which is key for good digestive health. It's also a plant-based source of omega-3 fatty acids and a big source of lignans. Lignans are those special *phytonutrients* (natural chemicals found in plants) that possess powerful antioxidant and anti-inflammatory properties.

You can buy flax in a few different ways: in whole seed form, already ground into powder form, or as flaxseed oil. All are available in local health food stores and some specialty supermarkets. Though flaxseed oil does have many health benefits, it lacks the valuable fiber of the seeds themselves because the fiber is separated from the oil during pressing. For best results, use ground flaxseed with the fiber intact, adding two tablespoons of ground flaxseed to your smoothie each day.

Store flaxseed oil and ground flaxseed in the refrigerator to keep them fresh. When flaxseed is processed into a powder or an oil, it becomes temperature-sensitive and turns rancid much more quickly if left at room temperature. If you buy it already ground, simply put it in the refrigerator after opening the package.

Coconut oil

The high percentage of lauric acid in coconut oil makes it a true healing food. Research has shown that *lauric acid* can increase the good high-density lipoprotein (HDL) cholesterol and actually decrease the bad low-density lipoprotein (LDL) cholesterol. Other studies indicate that coconut oil can boost metabolism, lower sugar cravings, and help people lose weight. Coconut oil is also known to contain powerful antimicrobial, antioxidant, antifungal, and antibacterial properties.

Coconut oil is naturally high in fat, which means it's a high-calorie food, so use it minimally. Just a tablespoon in your green smoothie per day gives you plenty of the healing power without too many extra calories. Search for coconut oil in the cooking oil section of your supermarket or find it in your local health food store.

Cinnamon

You may think of cinnamon as a common everyday spice, but it's actually a fantastic superfood. Cinnamon is known as a powerful anti-inflammatory and high-antioxidant food and contains calcium, manganese, and iron. It's particularly good for improving indigestion, reducing bloating, bettering circulation, and lowering blood sugar levels. Cinnamon also helps you heal from bacterial infections, improves heart health and brain function, fights off cancer cells, and relieves pain associated with arthritis.

You can find ground cinnamon in the normal spice section of your supermarket. Simply add a half teaspoon per day to your green smoothie.

Goji berries

Goji berries, also known as *wolfberries,* have been used in China as an herbal medicine and a healing food for more than 2,000 years. The goji berry is a complete source of protein — meaning it contains all eight essential amino acids — and has twice the amount of antioxidants as blueberries.

Goji berries are normally sold dried, either in whole form or powdered form. You can find whole versions at Chinese herbal shops and other forms at specialty food markets and online. If you're using the whole dried berries, soak them for at least one hour in water to rehydrate them before adding to your green smoothie. Add a tablespoon of goji berry powder or soaked goji berries to your smoothie.

Maca powder

Maca is a superfood that comes from the Andes Mountains in Peru. Health benefits of maca include reduced risk of prostate cancer, strengthened immune system, increased stamina, and improved memory. It's also said to be a natural stress reliever.

Other studies show that maca helps to balance hormones, decrease the effects of menopause, and even increase sex drive. If you're interested in a more amorous partner, try adding maca powder to his or her daily smoothie. You can thank me later!

Maca is a root vegetable and most commonly sold in powder form, although you can also find it in *tincture* (liquid) form. You can find maca online, at health food stores, and even some in pharmacies. Add one to two tablespoons of maca powder or 15 to 20 drops of maca tincture to your smoothie.

Choosing organic superfoods

If you should buy any one food organic, it's your superfood. Why? Currently, many food companies take advantage of the fact that not a lot of regulation governs the quality or ingredients used in superfood powders. If a superfood isn't 100 percent certified organic, it's allowed to have added fillers that include anything from rice powder to bran, oats, apple pectin, barley malt, large amounts of lecithin, and even added sugar. Essentially, manufacturers can pump a product full of fillers and include just a small amount of the expensive superfood ingredient. Of course, they still charge a high price, leaving the innocent consumer none the wiser. Not anymore!

Choose only 100 percent certified organic superfoods, and you get the highest quality ingredients with no added fillers. Here's a legal loophole: If the word *organic* is in name of the product but the product doesn't have the 100 percent certified organic seal, then it may not truly be organic. For example, there's nothing organic about a paper clip, but you could legally sell one as "My Organic Paper Clip" as long as you didn't include the seal. Be sure to look for the 100 percent certified organic seal pictured here. Yes, investing in the certified organic version of a superfood is more expensive, but spending a bit more as an investment in your health is worth it. Check for online sales, store coupons, or buy in bulk to save a bit of money.

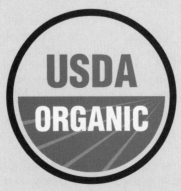

Graphic from www.fda.gov

Adding Other Supplements

You can use superfoods in general to boost your smoothie on an everyday basis. But sometimes you may want to add even more, especially if you start to feel under the weather and you want to prevent getting full-blown sick. Having some simple but powerful healing foods or supplements on hand gives you a natural medicine kit at home, ready to blend into an extra-healing green smoothie when needed.

Letting your food be your medicine

Hippocrates, the founder of modern medicine, once said, "Let food be thy medicine and medicine be thy food." That was back in 400 BC, but the saying still applies today. Yep, that Hippocrates knew his stuff. Using food as medicine is an ancient science, and every culture around the world has healing foods that people know to take when sick. Maybe your mom gave you chicken soup to recover from colds and flu as a kid. In India and China, they've been using turmeric and ginger to relieve fevers, colds, and intestinal problems for centuries. In the following sections, I show you some modern ways to blend healing foods into your green smoothies to help you recover more quickly and get back on your healthy feet.

Deciding when to use extras and what to use

As soon as you feel the first symptoms of a cold, sore throat, cough, or general malaise, try adding some of these healing supplements/foods to your green smoothie to give your immune system an extra boost. Combine that with plenty of water and rest and allow your body time to heal naturally.

For any extreme symptoms, high fever, or serious medical concerns, consulting a doctor is always best.

For cold and flu

If you feel a cold coming on or you're in the throes of a full-blown flu, add foods that are naturally high in vitamin C to your green smoothie. Fresh parsley, kale, pineapple, orange, lemon, papaya, kiwi, cantaloupe, and strawberries are all great options.

In addition, add some grapefruit seed extract (GSE) to your daily smoothie until you start feeling better. GSE is a powerful antiviral, antifungal, and anti-parasitic agent and often helps nip foreign invaders in the bud. Add 12 to 15 drops of grapefruit seed extract (GSE) for adults and 3 to 5 drops for children. Be sure to dilute the GSE in your smoothie and not drink it straight because it's strong stuff!

You can also add *echinacea* and *goldenseal,* natural herbs that are known to be powerful immune boosters. These herbs are easiest to add in a liquid or tincture form and are often sold together as one supplement combined. Add one dropper full of the liquid to a smoothie for adults. ***Note:*** Whether goldenseal is safe for children is unknown, so don't use this herbal combination in smoothies for kids.

For a sore throat, add fresh lemon, ginger, and manuka honey to your smoothie. This natural combo is perfectly safe for everyone, including children. Manuka honey is a special honey collected from the wild, uncultivated tea tree bush in New Zealand. It's pure, raw, natural, unpasteurized, and organic. Most importantly, manuka honey has amazing antibacterial properties. Add two tablespoons of fresh lemon juice, an inch-by-inch piece of fresh ginger, and two tablespoons of manuka honey with your other smoothie ingredients, blend, and drink.

For upset stomach

Anti-inflammatory foods such as fresh turmeric and fresh ginger are very helpful for an upset stomach. Add a small slice of each to your smoothie and blend until smooth.

Fresh banana and apple are good fruits to help calm an upset stomach. For nausea, you can add a small amount of fresh peppermint leaves or a little pure peppermint oil to your smoothie.

For migraine headache

Magnesium deficiency has been directly linked to migraines in a number of major studies, so putting magnesium-rich foods in your smoothie can provide relief. Magnesium is known as the relaxing mineral because it helps calm the nerves and release tension in muscles. Add pumpkin seeds, sunflower seeds, sesame seeds, flaxseed, spinach, kale, or Swiss chard to your smoothie to boost magnesium naturally. Raw, unsalted seeds are best.

Cayenne pepper can also help. It helps equalize blood pressure and thus relieves pressure in the head region. Add a dash of cayenne to your smoothie; if you can stand the taste, add a bit more.

If you suffer from nausea because of the migraine, try adding some fresh ginger or fresh peppermint leaves to your smoothie. (I discuss other nausea remedies in the preceding section.)

Figuring Out Which Liquids Are Best for Your Smoothie

Getting the perfect smoothie is all about adding the right liquid. You can add many types of liquids to a smoothie, and in this section I cover the most popular options and help you figure out which is best for you. Some common choices aren't actually as healthy as you may think.

Can or should you add coffee to a green smoothie, too? I've heard of people using coffee in their green smoothies, but I don't recommend it. For one, coffee is acid-forming, a characteristic that goes against the alkaline nature of the fruits and greens. Plus, I can't think of any reason to violate the taste of a smoothie with something as strong as coffee. If you need to drink coffee in the morning, make it organic and have a cup *after* you drink your green smoothie.

Hailing hydration: Water is best

The bottom line: Plain water is the simplest choice, but it's also the best! It's a natural liquid, free of chemical additives and thickening agents. It contains no fat, calories, or added sugars. It's easy to digest and naturally anti-inflammatory. It's also not expensive.

On a daily basis, most people don't drink enough water. The body needs water to stay hydrated and healthy. Chronic dehydration can lead to dry skin, constipation, bad breath, headaches, and low energy levels. Why not use your green smoothie to up your water intake? Ideally, filtered or bottled water is best.

Going cuckoo for coconut water

Coconut water isn't the same as coconut milk. *Coconut water* is the liquid found inside young green coconuts, and it tends to be sold in plastic containers rather than cans. Coconut water isn't made from coconut flesh, so it has a much lower fat content than coconut milk. (To compare, a cup of coconut milk has about 450 calories and almost 50 grams of fat, whereas a cup of coconut water has roughly 45 calories and less than a gram of fat. Head to the following section for more on coconut milk.)

Drinking coconut water is one of the hippest, newest diet trends since sliced bread. Some people call coconut water a superfood because of its antifungal, anti-parasitic, and antiviral properties.

Coconut water does contain electrolytes, sodium, and potassium, all of which help balance fluids after exercise, so on occasion, it can be a nice change from plain water in your smoothie.

Be sure to look for unsweetened varieties of coconut water so you aren't getting a bunch of added sugar. Some brands have 11 to 15 grams of sugar per serving. (An actual green coconut has roughly 6 grams of natural sugar per serving.) The ingredients should say "100 percent coconut water." Even better, buy the young green coconuts and open them yourself. That way, you're getting the freshest possible version without any added sugar, preservatives, or pasteurization. Some local health food stores and Asian markets sell fresh young green coconuts in the cold section of the store.

Getting the skinny on vegan milks

With the exception of water, any liquid that you add to your smoothie contains some form of additional calories. Most store-bought *vegan milks* (such as nut, rice, and soy milk) also have added sugar, flavorings, and/or chemical additives to create a smoother, creamier texture. They're not easy on the wallet, either. I personally don't think you need any vegan milks in your smoothie, but using one on occasion to shake things up is okay. On a daily basis, plain fresh water is your best choice.

- **Almond milk:** Store-bought almond milk can have added sugar and artificial flavors, neither of which is going to help you get any healthier. Always check the ingredients on the label before you buy to make sure the product is unsweetened and without chemical additives. Homemade almond milk is easy to make yourself, and you can add it to a smoothie for a good source of calcium, vitamin A, and vitamin D. As shown in Figure 6-1, to make fresh almond milk, soak raw, unsalted almonds overnight in water. The next day, rinse the almonds and then blend them with water until smooth. Use a cheesecloth to separate the fiber from the liquid. The liquid that's left is your homemade almond milk!

Even fresh homemade almond milk is stripped of fiber. You can still get all the valuable fiber and do less work by choosing an old-fashioned handful of raw almonds as an excellent healthy snack and opting for another liquid in your smoothie.

- **Coconut milk:** *Coconut milk* is the cream of grated coconut flesh and is usually sold in cans. It tends to be high in fat and often has added sugar, so it's very high in calories. It's a good option if you're trying to gain weight, but otherwise you should steer clear of coconut milk.

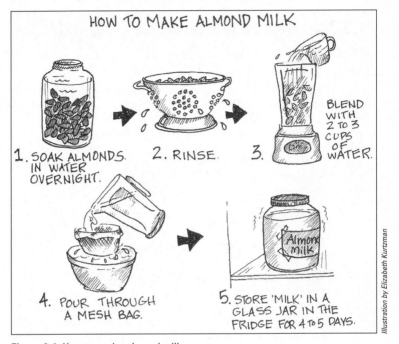

HOW TO MAKE ALMOND MILK

1. SOAK ALMONDS. IN WATER OVERNIGHT.

2. RINSE.

3. BLEND WITH 2 TO 3 CUPS OF WATER.

4. POUR THROUGH A MESH BAG.

5. STORE 'MILK' IN A GLASS JAR IN THE FRIDGE FOR 4 TO 5 DAYS.

Almond Milk

Illustration by Elizabeth Kurtzman

Figure 6-1: How to make almond milk.

✔ **Rice milk:** *Rice milk* is made from boiled rice, brown rice syrup, and brown rice starch. It's usually fortified with calcium or vitamin D, but manufacturers often also add thickening agents, sugar, flavorings, and artificial colorings to rice milk. The result is a high-sugar, high-carbohydrate drink with absolutely no fiber. You can better utilize rice by eating whole brown rice with the fiber and no added chemical ingredients and keeping the rice milks out of your blender.

✔ **Soy milk:** I can think of a lot of good reasons to pass on soy milk for your smoothies. They contain an additive called *carrageenan,* which is a thickening agent that increases inflammation, especially gastrointestinal inflammation. Flavored soy milks also contain artificial flavors and added sugar.

Of course, the other concern with soy milk is the genetic modification issue. More than 90 percent of soy in the United States is a genetically modified organism (GMO). That makes soy higher in certain proteins known to trigger food allergies and intolerances — especially in children, whose smaller bodies can't handle the high amounts of excess proteins. The other major issue with GMO foods is their direct link to infertility.

Knowing What to Leave out of Your Green Smoothie

When you see how easy throwing ingredients in the blender is, you may be tempted to start adding more — and more and more. But not everything you find in your fridge, freezer, or pantry should go into your green smoothies. Remember, the goal of the green smoothie is to make a healthy, nutrient-dense drink that boosts your vitamin and mineral reserve. Keep that goal in mind as you consider a few ingredients that are best left out.

Ditching dairy: Yogurt, milk, and cottage cheese

Whether or not dairy products are considered healthy is definitely a source of some controversy in the health and diet world. I'm not here to tell you to consume or not consume dairy products; that's a decision you should make on your own based on what feels best for you. I suggest that you keep dairy products out of your green smoothies.

Dairy products generate a lot of excess mucous through the process of digestion, and excess mucous can slow down digestion and absorption. Remember, the goal of drinking a green smoothie every day is to get more nutrients in your diet. If you add an ingredient that slows down absorption, you're losing a lot of the nutritional value of the smoothie. Why not keep your green smoothie dairy-free and allow your gut to absorb all its goodness?

Keeping your smoothie dairy-free also keeps the calorie count lower, and that's a good thing for anyone trying to achieve or maintain a healthy weight. If you choose to eat dairy products, that's okay; just eat them at another time of day in a separate meal or as a snack.

Refusing refined sugar

You're probably not surprised to read that today's diet, health, and medical experts recommend limiting refined sugar intake. Excess sugar in the diet can lead to a wide range of health problems, including obesity, heart disease, diabetes, and high blood pressure.

Even if you don't actually add sugar to your food, it's hidden in a lot of packaged foods such as Greek yogurt (especially the flavored kind), health drinks, cereals, condiments (such as ketchup), and even bottled "vitamin" water. Keep a sharp eye on the ingredients lists of products you put in your smoothie.

You absolutely don't need to add refined sugar to a green smoothie. You're only adding unnecessary calories devoid of any nutritional value. Besides, green smoothies already taste sweet from the natural sugars in fruit. And they're full of dietary fiber, which helps the body regulate sugar intake at a healthy, natural pace. Refer to Chapter 5 if you're still looking to sweeten up your smoothie; I show you healthy ways to do so with more fruits and other natural sweeteners.

Ignoring ice

Adding ice to a smoothie isn't the worst thing you can do, but it's not the best way to make a healthy smoothie, either. When you consume really cold or iced food, your stomach has to work extra hard just to heat the food back up inside your body. That weakens your digestive fire, and all those nutritious greens, high-fiber fruits, and powerful superfoods may not absorb properly. Digestion is slow, and indigestion can follow.

If you want a cool drink, blend with cold water instead of using ice. As an occasional treat on a hot day, you can add some frozen fruit to your smoothie, but take your time eating it. Let the smoothie warm up in your mouth a bit before swallowing, allowing the enzymes in your saliva to start the predigestive process in your mouth. As the ancient texts of Ayurvedic medicine say, "Drink your food and chew your drinks."

Putting the brakes on protein powders

Protein powders are proteins extracted from certain foods such as peas, soy, whey, or rice to make a highly concentrated dietary supplement. Consuming high concentrations of extracted proteins in powdered form is a relatively new diet trend. Certainly, these powders haven't been used by traditional cultures around the world for centuries like superfoods have. The danger in eating high concentrations of any food that isn't in its whole, natural form is that your body may not be able to handle it. Not to mention the fact that many protein powders contain synthetic chemicals, added sugar, and artificial flavorings.

Newer evidence shows that using protein powders can increase your risk of kidney disease and kidney stones. Some studies even suggest that some protein powders are contaminated with heavy metals. High-protein diets have been linked to an increased risk of osteoporosis and heart disease. Because these powders are so new, it may take some time for all the evidence to come out. In the meantime, why take a risk?

 I suggest that you avoid protein powders and get your protein from real, whole food such as organic eggs and meat. Of course, you can find plenty of natural protein in vegan and vegetarian whole foods such as seeds, nuts, spirulina, green leafy vegetables, alfalfa sprouts, sunflower sprouts, and legumes.

If you decide to use protein powders, choose 100 percent certified organic and look for a reputable brand. Definitely avoid any cheap generic supplements covered with lots of weight loss or muscle-building claims.

 Even within the better brands, you should always avoid certain types of protein powders. Check the ingredients before buying; if the product contains pea protein, yeast extract, natural flavors, and/or artificial flavors, walk away. Pea protein and yeast extract are additives with a high glutamate content and can cause headaches, insomnia, anxiety, and restlessness in people who are sensitive to monosodium glutamate (MSG). Natural flavors can contain hidden forms of MSG, and artificial flavors can definitely contain MSG. None of those items makes for a healthy smoothie ingredient. When in doubt, leave it out!

Chapter 7

Adjusting Smoothie Ingredients to Suit Your Taste

In This Chapter

▶ Tailoring your smoothie to your palate

▶ Knowing what to do with the fruit skins, seeds, and stems

E*veryone's taste buds are different. Some people prefer sweet, while others like bitter, savory, or even sour. The most important thing in making your green smoothies is that they taste good to you. If they don't taste good, you're not going to want to drink them. If you don't want to drink them, you won't keep making them. And if you don't keeping making them . . . well, you get the picture. You have to actually like your smoothies if you're going to realistically keep them as a healthy habit for life!

In this chapter, I share advice on tweaking the taste and texture of your smoothies to find what you like best. I also discuss including different parts of your fruits and vegetables, like peels and stems, and how those additions can affect taste.

Adding Greens, Fruit, or Water to Get Your Smoothie Just Right

Raw green leafy vegetables tend to have a bitter taste from their high mineral content — and that's a good thing — but the bitterness takes some getting used to. Fresh fruits tend to have a sweet taste, and some fruits (like green apple) have a slightly sour taste. The key to making a good green smoothie is being able to balance out the flavors so it tastes just right.

Use the recipes in Parts III and IV of this book as a guideline for what ingredients to add, but allow your taste buds to get a vote on the final outcome. Dip a spoon in your blended smoothie (with the blender turned off, of course) and have a quick taste. If your fruit wasn't ripe enough, it may taste a bit bland. If you added too many greens, it may seem too bitter. Or the texture may be too thick or soupy. Fear not! Part of the learning curve in becoming a smoothie expert is understanding how to adjust the flavor and consistency to make a smoothie that tastes good to you, and that's what I break down in the following sections. Green smoothies may look a bit scary at first from the unusual green color, but they can and should taste delicious!

If you have different palates within the same household, you can adjust your smoothies to order. I personally like more greens in my smoothie, so I make my boyfriend's smoothie first with the standard amount of greens in the recipe. I pour him a glass and then add more greens into what's left to make my extra-green green smoothie.

When you first start making green smoothies, you may land on a favorite combination of fruits and greens and find yourself making the same smoothie every day because you're comfortable with the recipe you have. But don't be afraid to experiment with fruits and greens that you've never eaten before. More variety in your diet means more minerals and nutrients, and that makes for a healthier you. You don't know how to cook Swiss chard? It doesn't matter when you're putting it in a green smoothie; you still get all the nutritional value! Take advantage of how easy green smoothies are to make. Experiment with new ingredients and have fun with it.

When to add more greens

Include more greens to your smoothie if it tastes too sweet. The bitter taste of green leafy veggies helps balance the sweet flavor of the fruits. A smoothie can be sweet from using naturally sweet fruits such as pineapple, mango, guava, passion fruit, or melon. Fruit that is really ripe or overripe can also make a smoothie taste sweet. Of course, a sweet-tasting green smoothie is okay, but if it tastes too sweet and you don't enjoy the sweetness, then I suggest that you add more greens.

Large leafy greens such as kale, Swiss chard, collard greens, bok choy, beet greens, and romaine lettuce tend to be the most bitter. Smaller leaves such as watercress, baby spinach, parsley, and cilantro have a milder taste. Celery leaves have their own unique flavor that some people really don't like. Keep that in mind when adding more greens to your smoothie.

If your smoothie tastes too sweet, add more fresh leafy greens or more fresh lemon or lime juice. To adjust the flavor, add a small amount of greens, blend, and taste. If it's still too sweet, add more greens, but again in small amounts. Add no more than ½ cup of additional greens at a time. For fresh lemon or lime, add ¼ of a fresh lemon or lime squeezed at a time. You can always add more, but you can't take the extra out if you add too much.

Add more greens to your smoothie if you

✔ Enjoy bitter flavor more than sweet

✔ Are sensitive or intolerant to fruit sugars

✔ Don't eat greens in your normal daily diet

✔ Crave the taste of greens

✔ Are healing from injury or illness and want more chlorophyll and nutrients for faster recovery

When to add more fruit

Fruit is an important ingredient in a green smoothie recipe because the sweet taste of fruit helps to balance the bitter taste of greens. Fruit also adds more water content, enzymes, and fiber, all of which make the smoothie easier to digest and absorb.

Ripe fruit has a sweeter taste than unripe fruit. Think of the difference in taste between a green, unripe banana and a brown, overripe banana. Unripe fruit is starchy, tough, and sometimes bitter. As fruits ripen, the amount of starch decreases and the sugar content increases. Overripe fruit can start to oxidize, developing brown spots where the fruit is going bad, and occasionally mold even starts to appear on the outer skin. You don't want to eat that! Ideally, you should use fruit that is perfectly ripe — not too soft and without any large brown spots. Get tips on how to save your overripe fruit by freezing it for later use in Chapters 3 and 5. If a fruit is bruised, simply cut away the brown parts and use only the ripe portion.

If your smoothie doesn't taste sweet because you added unripe fruit, adding *more* unripe fruit won't sweeten it. In that case, you can add a tablespoon of raw honey, a teaspoon of stevia powder, or one medjool date to sweeten up the taste. Chapter 5 has more information on the different sweeteners you can use in a smoothie.

If you've taste-tested your smoothie and find it's not sweet enough, double-check your recipe and make sure you added the fruit initially called for before you start trying to adjust the taste. Believe it or not, you can easily make a green smoothie and actually forget to add the fruit!

Fruits such as banana, mango, pineapple, papaya, watermelon, and melon are very sweet and are good choices to help hide the bitter taste of greens. Sweet fruits are also great for hiding the strong taste of certain superfoods, such as spirulina and chlorella powder (which I discuss in Chapter 6). Lower glycemic index (GI) fruits such as strawberries, blueberries, and grapefruit tend to be less sweet. For more information on glycemic index, refer to the sidebar in Chapter 13.

Add an additional half cup of sweet fruit such as banana, apple, or pineapple to balance the taste if your smoothie is too bitter. Add the fruit, blend again, and then have a taste. You can add one or two medjool dates or a tablespoon of raw honey to heighten the sweet flavor if your smoothie tastes sour or even bland.

Add more fruit to your smoothie if you

- Enjoy sweet flavor more than bitter
- Are transitioning off refined sugar and/or wheat
- Want to hide the algae taste of spirulina powder
- Feel hungry between meals
- Suffer from a sluggish colon or constipation

When to add more water

The texture of your smoothie is also a matter of personal taste. Some people enjoy a thick green smoothie and actually prefer to eat it with a spoon, like a soup. Others prefer a much more drinkable or juice-like consistency. As you try new recipes, you can experiment with different textures and choose what works best for you.

If your smoothie seems too thick, add half a cup of water and blend again. If you still see green leaves that haven't been broken down by the blender blades, add another cup of water and blend again. If the smoothie is too watery, add two tablespoons of ground flaxseed and blend again.

Don't forget to put the lid of the blender back on as you adjust the taste and blend again; otherwise, you may end up with green smoothie on your ceiling!

Incorporating the Right Parts of Your Produce

The best thing about using a blender to make smoothies is that everything gets broken down. No one will notice if you accidentally squeeze in a few lemon seeds, add the apple stem, or throw in old, wilted celery leaves. But do you actually want to use those ingredients? Are they good for you, or do they take away nutritional value?

Debating skin-on produce

The outer skins of fruits and vegetables contain valuable minerals and are especially high in silicon. Known as the "beauty mineral," *silicon* is the best mineral for strong nails and hair and glowing skin. Silicon is also an essential mineral, along with calcium, for the growth and maintenance of joints and bones.

A deficiency in silicon can result in the following:

- Thinning hair
- Brittle nails
- Formation of wrinkles
- General aging of the skin

That's a pretty good advertisement to start eating those apple skins! But wait; not all fruit skins are equal.

Fruits that aren't organic may be sprayed with pesticides and/or coated in wax to give them a shiny, fresh look. The wax coating actually seals in the pesticides, making them virtually impossible to remove.

The other problem with not peeling your fruits, organic or not, is that you can miss a bruised or rotten part of the fruit. Have you ever cut an apple or pear in half and discovered that everything was brown and mushy inside? That's no fun, and it certainly doesn't taste good or make your smoothie nutritious. Regardless of whether you peel, always cut your fruits before putting them in the blender; that way, you can slice away any bad parts and leave only the fresh bits to blend.

Certain fruits such as papaya, mango, pineapple, avocado, banana, melon, grapefruit, orange, and lemon have a thick, bitter, or inedible skin, and you don't want those peels in a smoothie. Adding small amounts of lemon rind for taste is okay, but don't use the whole lemon skin.

Apples, pears, peaches, apricots, plums, grapes, kiwis, cucumbers, and tomatoes all have edible skins that you can add to your smoothie with the fruit, even if they're not organic. Just wash everything well first. Refer to Chapter 3 for instructions on how to wash your greens and fruit. Organic with the skin is always the best choice because those fruits have no dangerous pesticides or wax coating; they can even contain more minerals than non-organic fruits because they're grown in higher quality, more nutrient-dense soil.

Using or losing fruit cores and seeds

Whether to add the core of fruits and/or the seeds of a fruit is a simple matter of taste. The stems of fruits like grapes or apples don't contain any real nutritional value, so you can discard them. Seeds can have nutritional benefits but tend to have a bitter flavor; if you aren't into bitter smoothies, you're better off leaving out all the seeds and going with a smoothie that tastes good because a good tasting smoothie is one you'll drink every day.

Honeydew melon and cantaloupe seeds are high in protein and are full of powerful antioxidants along with vitamin E, magnesium, phosphorous, and potassium. Definitely add these seeds to your green smoothie! Watermelon seeds contain zinc, iron, and protein, so including them in your smoothie is a good idea as well.

Citrus seeds such as lemon, lime, and orange are edible, but they tend to be bitter. If you don't mind or don't notice the bitter taste, then adding them to your smoothie is fine. Strawberry seeds and blackberry seeds are okay too. Blackberry seeds in particular are rich in protein, carotenoids, and omega-3 fatty acids.

Apple seeds contain *amygdalin,* a substance that produces cyanide through the process of digestion. This same substance also occurs naturally in apricot, cherry, peach, pear, and plum pits and seeds. Blending up one or two apples plus a pear, seeds and all, isn't going to do any damage, but you're still probably better off cutting away the core and throwing out the pits, adding only the fruit to your smoothie. I don't recommend large-scale consumption of any of these seeds.

The avocado seed contains high amounts of potassium and powerful antioxidants; you can blend them, but only if you have a high-power blender such as a Vitamix. Large seeds or pits like avocado are just too big for the small motor in a standard household blender. Avoid mango pits altogether because they haven't been found to be edible in a raw form.

Tossing stems and leaves in or out

When using small leafy greens such as fresh parsley, baby spinach, watercress, or celery leaves, add the whole leaves with the stems. Not only does it save you time spent cutting away each small stem, but you also get more minerals, chlorophyll, and fiber simply by eating more of the leafy greens in each smoothie.

If you're using big leafy greens such as kale, Swiss chard, or collard greens in your smoothie, you can either cut away the large stems or add them to your smoothie. The larger stems contain added minerals and chlorophyll, but they have a really bitter taste. If you're new to making smoothies, you may want to avoid using the big stems because that extra bitter taste may turn you off. Over time, as you get used to the bitter taste of greens, you can always add some green stems.

The motor in your blender is also a determining factor in whether you can use thick, leafy stems in your smoothie. Generally speaking, if the motor is 700 watts or greater, the blender should be able to handle blending thicker, larger leafy stems. If it's less than 700 watts, those big leaves will stress the motor, and your blender may not survive too long. If your blender motor is less than 700 watts, cut the large stems off and set them aside. If you have a juicer, you can save the stems for juicing later. Otherwise they can be discarded or put in a compost bin (more on composting below). Be nice to your blender, and your blender will be nice to you!

You can actually use strawberry greens, beet greens, radish greens, and parsley and cilantro stems in your green smoothie instead of throwing them away. I keep a bag of "leftover" greens in my fridge that I collect over the course of a few days or a week. This collection is my go-to bag of greens for my smoothies, especially if I happen to run out of other fresh greens.

Making use of leftover ingredients

You've made a delicious-tasting green smoothie, and you have a blender on standby for the next healthy creation. You may also have a small pile of leftovers: apple cores, some kale stems, lemon skins, and maybe some tomato stems, wilted celery, or celery ends that didn't make the cut.

If you have a juicer at home, you can use certain leftovers in a juice. Celery ends, wilted greens, kale stems, large leafy stems, and parsley or cilantro stems are all perfect ingredients for a healthy green juice. (***Note:*** A green juice is different from a green smoothie. Refer to Chapter 2 for details on juicers and how to make a green juice.) I keep one leftover bag in my fridge just for juice. Once a week, I make a "whatever's in the fridge" juice. I clean out all the older fruit and veggies, and that's when I use my leftover bag, too. I toss all the ingredients in the juicer, usually adding some ginger and lemon to brighten the taste, and I toast to good health and to not wasting any valuable, fresh food!

If you have a compost bin, you can add your green smoothie leftovers to it. The only leftovers you shouldn't compost are citrus peels and garlic and ginger skins. Citrus isn't actually bad for the compost, but it takes a long time to break down. Even if you grind it up in your blender before you toss it in the bin, it takes longer than any other food to decompose and slows down the overall compost time. The bugs and worms in the bin have a bit of an aversion to citrus, and they don't like garlic or ginger either (because both are antiparasitic foods).

Composting provides you with rich organic matter that does wonders to improve the quality of your garden soil. Your garden plants and landscape will grow healthier and stronger thanks to the mineral-rich soil. Check out *Composting For Dummies* by Cathy Cromell (Wiley) to find out about composting at home.

Smoothies: Snack or meal replacement?

You can use your smoothie as a snack, as the first course before a meal, or as the meal itself. Initially, you may not be ready to make it a total meal replacement, and that's okay. In that case, I recommend that you drink your smoothie first. You can satisfy whatever room you have leftover with your normal meal. If you try leaving your smoothie until after the meal, you may just unconsciously fill up on refined carbohydrates or other empty calories, and before you know it, you have no room or desire to drink any healthy anything. Drinking the smoothie first is a surefire way to drink a smoothie every day; with any luck, you'll feel so full and satiated from the fiber and nutrients in the smoothie that you naturally won't want any more food.

The other option is to start by having green smoothies as an afternoon or evening snack. That's definitely a better choice than the old go-to processed foods or comfort snacks. Eating healthy snacks between meals can make you less hungry at mealtime, which means you eat less. Overall, you still get the same results as the replacement meal option. Just find the best routine that works for you.

Part III
Green Smoothies for Every Day

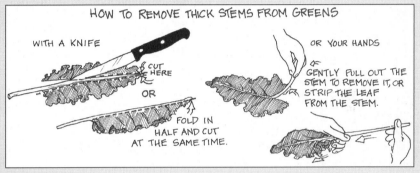

Illustration by Elizabeth Kurtzman

Head to www.dummies.com/extras/greensmoothies for a week's worth of green smoothie information, including a shopping list and menus.

In this part . . .

✔ Get blending with green smoothie recipe ideas for morning, noon, and night — or any time of day, because you're free to enjoy any smoothie whenever you want!

✔ Find out how to prepare your ingredients in advance and what to do with the leftovers so that a tasty, nutritious green smoothie is never far away.

✔ Blend up green smoothie recipes that kids will love, from baby to toddler to teenager, and find out the best ingredients to use based on age.

Chapter 8

Morning Green Smoothies

*B*reakfast is an important meal because it provides your body with fuel in the form of food. If you find yourself in a time crunch every morning, this chapter is for you; each recipe takes less than 5 minutes to prepare and can be made the night before, so the mayhem of the morning rush is no longer an excuse to skip breakfast! Simply store a premade smoothie in the fridge in a sealed container overnight and grab it and go in the morning. Good nutritional health doesn't get much easier than that!

This chapter presents recipes that are perfect for a healthy breakfast. Each smoothie contains valuable fiber from the fruits and greens and doesn't have too much fat. That way, the smoothie is easy to digest and provides you with more energy for the day. In fact, after drinking one of these smoothies every morning, you may find that you no longer even need a cup of coffee.

The Bee and Berry Power smoothie in this chapter calls for bee pollen, which you should leave out if you're allergic to pollen or to bees. Even if you don't have one of these allergies, before including that ingredient in a smoothie flip to Chapter 6 for info on how to determine whether you're sensitive to consuming bee pollen.

If you exercise first thing in the morning and want a heartier smoothie for your first meal of the day, turn to Chapter 9 for midday smoothies you can substitute for breakfast.

Getting a Healthy Start to a Good Day

What better way to start the day than with your healthiest meal first? Drinking a green smoothie in the morning gives you the best chance to make better food choices for the rest of the day. Just imagine how you feel after a heavy cooked breakfast of bacon, eggs, toast, and fried potatoes. Do you really want to have a light salad after that, or do you continue to crave carbs and fat all day?

If you do things right from the starting gate, you naturally want to keep feeling good all day. From there, making better food choices is so much easier. Without even thinking about it, you find yourself instinctively gravitating toward more good food. When your body starts getting all the nutrients it needs, you won't feel the need to snack or overeat, either.

Preparing smoothie ingredients in advance

To save time in the morning, you can prepare fresh fruits and greens for your green smoothie the night before. Just try to use prepared ingredients within 24 hours. Follow these tips:

- Wash fruits and greens the night before, or better yet, as soon as you bring them home from the store. Find more details on how to clean your produce in Chapter 3.

- Chop up fruits such as pineapple or kiwi and store them in a sealed glass container in the fridge overnight. You can also peel oranges and store them in a zip-top bag.

- Store your superfoods and powders together in one area of your refrigerator so you can find them quickly.

- Put your smoothie container on the counter next to your blender so everything is ready to go first thing in the morning. If you see the blender sitting out and waiting to be used, you're much more likely to make that smoothie!

- If you're really not a morning person, go to Plan B: Make your smoothie the night before and store it in the fridge. Just don't forget to grab it on your way out the door!

Pineapple Coconut Breeze

Prep time: 3 min • **Blending time:** 2 min • **Yield:** 3 servings

Ingredients	Directions
1 orange, peeled and seeded	**1** Combine all ingredients except the kale in the blender and secure the lid.
1 cup pineapple chunks	
2 ripe bananas, peeled	**2** Starting at low speed and gradually increasing toward high, blend the ingredients for 1 minute or until the mixture contains no visible pieces of fruit.
2 teaspoons spirulina powder	
1 tablespoon acai powder	
1 tablespoon ground flaxseed	
2 cups coconut water	**3** Remove and discard the stems of the kale (see Figure 8-1). Add the kale leaves and blend again at medium speed for 30 seconds, gradually increasing the speed to high.
3 large kale leaves	
	4 Blend on high speed for another 15 to 30 seconds or until the entire mixture is smooth.
	5 Pour the smoothie into three glasses and enjoy!

Per serving: Calories 198 (From Fat 18); Fat 2g (Saturated 0.5g); Cholesterol 0mg; Sodium 205mg; Carbohydrate 43g (Dietary Fiber 7g); Protein 4g.

Tip: If you don't have coconut water, use 1½ cups of water plus 2 tablespoons of coconut oil instead.

Vary It! Try fresh papaya instead of pineapple. If you don't have access to tropical fruits, swap out the pineapple for kiwi or grapes.

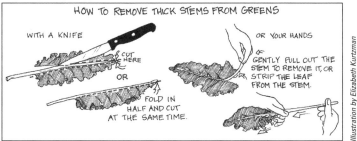

Figure 8-1: Techniques for removing stems from greens.

Mango Goji Delight

Prep time: 25 min • **Blending time:** 2 min • **Yield:** 2 servings

Ingredients	Directions
2 tablespoons dried goji berries	*1* Place the goji berries in a bowl with ¼ cup of room temperature water. Place in the fridge to soak for at least 20 minutes or overnight.
1 ripe mango	
1 ripe banana, peeled	
2 tablespoons ground flaxseed	*2* Peel the mango and cut the flesh away from the stone.
¼ cup fresh lime juice	
1½ cups water	*3* Combine the goji berries, mango, banana, flaxseed, lime juice, and water in the blender and secure the lid.
1 cup parsley, loosely packed	
1 cup baby spinach, loosely packed	*4* Starting at low speed and gradually increasing toward high, blend the ingredients for 1 minute or until smooth.
	5 Add the parsley and spinach and blend again at medium speed for 45 seconds, gradually increasing the speed to high.
	6 Pour the smoothie into two glasses and serve.

Per serving: Calories 200 (From Fat 36); Fat 4g (Saturated 0.5g); Cholesterol 0mg; Sodium 45mg; Carbohydrate 41g (Dietary Fiber 7g); Protein 5g.

Tip: For plumper, more flavorful goji berries, soak the dried berries in 1 cup of water overnight and use the water from soaking as a replacement for 1 cup of water in the recipe.

Vary It! In winter, use dried goji berries. In warmer months, replace them with fresh, in-season berries, such as raspberries, blackberries, or strawberries. For fresh berries, you can increase the amount to ½ cup.

Apple Cinnamon Joy

Prep time: 25 min • **Blending time:** 2 min • **Yield:** 2 servings

Ingredients	Directions
4 tablespoons chia seeds	**1** Place the chia seeds in a bowl with 1 cup of room temperature water. Place in the fridge to soak for at least 20 minutes or overnight.
2 red apples	
1 Medjool date, pitted	
1 ripe banana, peeled	**2** Cut the apples and remove the core, keeping the skin intact. Cut into quarters.
¼ teaspoon ground cinnamon	
1 cup water	**3** Add the chia seeds with soaking water, apples, date, banana, cinnamon, and additional water to the blender and secure the lid.
1 cup baby spinach, loosely packed	
1 cup watercress, loosely packed	**4** Starting at low speed and gradually increasing toward high, blend the ingredients for 1 minute or until the mixture contains no visible pieces of fruit.
	5 Add the spinach and watercress and blend again at medium speed for 45 seconds, gradually increasing the speed to high.
	6 Pour the smoothie into two glasses and serve.

Per serving: Calories 266 (From Fat 54); Fat 6g (Saturated 0.5g); Cholesterol 0mg; Sodium 24mg; Carbohydrate 55g (Dietary Fiber 12g); Protein 5g.

Tip: If you don't have chia seeds, use 4 tablespoons of ground flaxseed instead and increase the water to 2 cups.

Vary It! For a slightly different taste, add a pinch of ground cloves, ground cardamom, or 1 to 2 teaspoons of vanilla extract. Or instead of cinnamon, use ¼ teaspoon of ground nutmeg.

Bee and Berry Power

Prep time: 3 min • **Blending time:** 2 min • **Yield:** 2 servings

Ingredients	Directions
⅔ cup raspberries	*1* Combine all the ingredients except the Swiss chard in the blender and secure the lid.
⅔ cup halved strawberries, stems and leaves removed	
2 ripe bananas, peeled	*2* Starting at low speed and gradually increasing toward high, blend the ingredients for 1 minute or until the mixture contains no visible pieces of fruit.
1 tablespoon raw honey	
2 tablespoons hemp seeds	
1 tablespoon bee pollen (omit if allergic)	*3* Remove and discard the stems of the Swiss chard (see Figure 8-1). Add the Swiss chard leaves and blend again at medium speed for 30 seconds, gradually increasing the speed to high.
1 tablespoon coconut oil	
2 cups water	
4 large Swiss chard leaves	
	4 Blend on high speed for another 15 to 30 seconds or until the entire mixture is smooth.
	5 Pour the smoothie into two glasses and enjoy!

Per serving: Calories 343 (From Fat 135); Fat 15g (Saturated 15g); Cholesterol 0mg; Sodium 48mg; Carbohydrate 50g (Dietary Fiber 9g); Protein 9g.

Tip: Buy berries fresh and in season. When they're on sale, buy extra amounts to freeze and use throughout the winter. Wash the berries and remove any stems before freezing. Store them in zip-top bags in the freezer.

Tip: You can use either shelled raw hemp seeds or ground hemp seed. Use the same amount for either option.

Vary It! Use blueberries or blackberries instead of strawberries or raspberries.

Ginger Lemon Zinger

Prep time: 3 min • **Blending time:** 2 min • **Yield:** 3 servings

Ingredients	Directions
1 red apple	*1* Cut the apple and pear and remove the cores, keeping the skin intact. Cut the flesh into quarters.
1 ripe pear	
1 cup red or green grapes	
1 ripe banana, peeled	*2* Add all the ingredients except the kale to the blender and secure the lid.
2 tablespoons ground flaxseed	
½-inch piece fresh ginger (peeled)	*3* Starting at low speed and gradually increasing toward high, blend the ingredients for 1 minute or until the mixture contains no visible pieces of fruit.
¼ cup fresh lemon juice	
1½ cups water	
4 small or 2 large kale leaves	*4* Remove and discard the stems of the kale (see Figure 8-1). Add the kale leaves and blend again at medium speed for 30 seconds, gradually increasing the speed to high.
	5 Blend on high speed for another 15 to 30 seconds or until the entire mixture is smooth.
	6 Pour the smoothie into three glasses and serve.

Per serving: Calories 191 (From Fat 27); Fat 3g (Saturated 0g); Cholesterol 0mg; Sodium 16mg; Carbohydrate 44g (Dietary Fiber 6g); Protein 3g.

Tip: If you don't have fresh ginger, use ¼ teaspoon of ground ginger instead.

Vary It! Boost the nutritional value of this smoothie by adding 1 tablespoon of chlorella powder, 1 teaspoon of wheatgrass powder, or 1 teaspoon of spirulina powder in addition to the fresh greens.

What to do with the leftovers

Leftover smoothies make for an excellent afternoon snack! Put any extra smoothie in a sealed container and take it to work or school to drink later. Store it in the refrigerator until you're ready to drink it. For taste and freshness, I recommend drinking smoothies within two days of blending.

If you're really keen to share your leftovers, try giving some green smoothie to your dog. Yes, you can! I've given green smoothies to dogs on many occasions. Admittedly, they don't all like it, but some really do. Just avoid giving your dog any smoothies that contain cacao powder because any form of chocolate is not recommended for dogs.

Chapter 9

Midday Green Smoothies

In This Chapter

▶ Taking advantage of your natural digestive rhythm

▶ Satisfying smoothies for a lunch or snack

Are you so flat-out busy during the day that you simply don't have time to eat lunch? You don't even have time to chew, so you skip lunch only to arrive home later, completely drained and starving, and spend the next couple of hours eating everything in sight. Not anymore! Sipping on a smoothie midday is the way to go. Let the blender do the chewing for you! Just take slow sips and keep plowing through your day. You feel more satisfied and less drained, and you're able to make better food choices when you get home. In this chapter, you explore the convenient and easy ways to enjoy a healthy lunch or afternoon smoothie snack.

 WARNING!

The Pineapple Mango Coco-Yum smoothie in this chapter calls for bee pollen, which you should leave out if you're allergic to pollen or to bees. Even if you don't have one of these allergies, before including that ingredient in a smoothie check out Chapter 6 for important information on how to determine whether you're sensitive to consuming bee pollen.

Getting That Afternoon Energy Boost

Because your digestive fire is most active in the middle of the day, you have more energy to digest heavier foods at your midday meal. That's why the recipes in this chapter contain healthy fats such as avocado, nuts, or seeds. Not only do these ingredients make the smoothies taste thicker and creamier, but they also make you feel fuller. The goal is twofold: give you enough energy to get through the day without feeling any afternoon lull and leave you feeling satisfied enough to not snack on junk food later.

If you're someone who tends to crave a chocolate or sugar fix every afternoon, then a green smoothie for lunch is definitely right for you. Remember, a high fiber diet has been proven to help in stabilizing blood sugars. You can clean out your old chocolate bar drawer now because you won't need it anymore!

Because green smoothies stay fresh for up to 48 hours in the fridge, you can easily make your smoothie the night before or first thing in the morning like you would a brown-bag lunch.

Nuts, nut butter, or nut milk?

What's the difference among nuts, nut butter, and nut milk? Well, nuts are a whole food; *nut butters* are nuts that have been ground into a paste; and *nut milks* are a liquid drink made from soaking the nuts, blending with water, and then separating the fiber from the liquid with a cheesecloth. (Find out how to make almond milk at home in Chapter 6.) But the form of the food is only one thing to consider; you also have to decide whether to go raw or roasted.

Raw nuts are in their most natural and least processed form, and they still contain all their original, valuable enzymes. Roasted nuts are heated to high temperatures in the roasting process, which leaves all enzymes destroyed. Not only that, but roasted nuts often contain added salt and even monosodium glutamate (MSG), making them a less-than-healthy choice. Nut butters come in raw and roasted varieties depending on what kind of nut goes into them. Raw nut butters are a healthier choice than regular nut butters because the nuts in raw nut butter are still raw with the enzymes intact. Make sure you choose one without added oils or refined sugar, too. Raw nut butters may have a heftier price tag, but they're worth it.

In Chapter 6, I explain what's in nut milks and why I'm not a fan of store-bought nut milks. You can make homemade nut milks, but if you're short on time, my vote goes to raw nuts or raw nut butters.

Banana Kiwi Bliss

Prep time: 3 min • **Blending time:** 2 min • **Yield:** 2 servings

Ingredients	Directions
2 kiwis, peeled	*1* Combine the kiwi, avocado, banana, spirulina, flaxseed, orange juice, and water in the blender and secure the lid.
½ avocado, peeled and pitted (see Figure 9-1)	
1 ripe banana, peeled	*2* Starting at low speed and gradually increasing toward high, blend the ingredients for 45 seconds or until the mixture contains no visible pieces of fruit.
1 teaspoon spirulina powder	
1 tablespoon ground flaxseed	
1 cup fresh orange juice	
1 cup water	*3* Add the greens and spinach and blend again at medium speed for 30 seconds, gradually increasing the speed to high. Blend on high speed for another 15 to 30 seconds or until the entire mixture is smooth.
1 cup chopped parsnip greens or beet greens, stems removed	
1 cup baby spinach, loosely packed	
	4 Pour the smoothie into two glasses and enjoy!

Per serving: Calories 243 (From Fat 63); Fat 7g (Saturated 1g); Cholesterol 0mg; Sodium 93mg; Carbohydrate 43g (Dietary Fiber 9g); Protein 5g.

Tip: You should be able to find parsnip greens at most supermarkets. Beet greens are the green leaves attached to beets, and yes, you can use them in a green smoothie! If you can't find either of those items, just use an extra cup of baby spinach (for a total of 2 cups) instead.

Vary It! Instead of kiwi, try 1 cup of fresh pineapple. If the smoothie tastes too bitter to you, omit the spirulina, or check out Chapter 7 for more ways to adjust the taste to your liking.

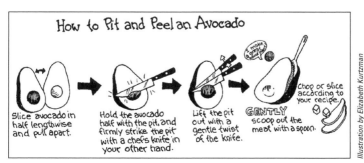

Figure 9-1: How to peel and pit an avocado.

Peaches and Green

Prep time: 3 min • **Blending time:** 2 min • **Yield:** 2 servings

Ingredients	Directions
2 ripe peaches	*1* Cut the peaches and remove the pit, keeping the skin intact. Cut the flesh into quarters.
1 ripe banana, peeled	
²⁄₃ cup halved strawberries, stems and leaves removed	*2* Combine all the ingredients except the kale in the blender and secure the lid.
3 tablespoons raw almond butter	
2 tablespoons coconut oil	*3* Starting at low speed and gradually increasing toward high, blend the ingredients for 45 seconds or until the mixture contains no visible pieces of fruit.
1 tablespoon raw honey	
1½ cups water	
4 large kale leaves	*4* Remove and discard the stems of the kale (see Figure 8-1). Loosely tear the kale into smaller pieces (precision isn't important) to make it easier to add to the blender. Add the kale leaves and blend again at medium speed for 30 seconds, gradually increasing the speed to high. Blend on high speed for another 15 to 30 seconds or until the entire mixture is smooth.
	5 Pour the smoothie into two glasses and enjoy!

Per serving: Calories 439 (From Fat 252); Fat 28g (Saturated 13g); Cholesterol 0mg; Sodium 21mg; Carbohydrate 48g (Dietary Fiber 8g); Protein 9g.

Tip: You can use coconut water instead of water in this recipe for even more coconut flavor. If you don't have raw almond butter, you can replace it with 8 raw almonds.

Tip: If you can't get fresh peaches (for example, in winter months), then it's okay to use frozen peaches as a replacement. Use 1 cup of frozen peaches to replace 2 fresh peaches.

Vary It! Use nectarines instead of peaches or raspberries instead of strawberries.

Candy Apple Delight

Prep time: 3 min • **Blending time:** 2 min • **Yield:** 2 servings

Ingredients	Directions
2 Granny Smith apples	*1* Cut the apples and remove the core, keeping the skin intact. Cut the flesh into quarters.
1 ripe banana, peeled	
2 Medjool dates, pitted	
3 tablespoons tahini	*2* Combine all the ingredients except the collard greens in the blender and secure the lid.
2 tablespoons hemp seeds	
1½ cups water	
4 large collard green leaves	*3* Starting at low speed and gradually increasing toward high, blend the ingredients for 30 to 45 seconds or until the mixture contains no visible pieces of fruit.
	4 Remove and discard the stems of the collard greens. Chop or tear the collard green leaves into smaller pieces (precision isn't important). Add the leaves and blend again at medium speed for 30 seconds, gradually increasing the speed to high. Blend on high speed for another 30 seconds or until the entire mixture is smooth.
	5 Pour the smoothie into two glasses and enjoy!

Per serving: Calories 491 (From Fat 171); Fat 19g (Saturated 11g); Cholesterol 0mg; Sodium 16mg; Carbohydrate 73g (Dietary Fiber 12g); Protein 12g.

Tip: You can usually find *tahini,* a paste made from sesame seeds, in health food stores or gourmet supermarkets. Look for it in the peanut butter and jam section or in the ethnic section of your local store.

Vary It! Instead of tahini, you can use raw almond butter. You can also replace the banana with ½ avocado (peeled and pitted) for a slightly different taste.

Cacao Maca Super Boost

Prep time: 5 min • **Blending time:** 2 min • **Yield:** 2 servings

Ingredients	*Directions*
1 orange, peeled and seeded	*1* Combine all the ingredients except the spinach in the blender and secure the lid.
1 ripe banana, peeled	
½ teaspoon vanilla extract	*2* Starting at low speed and gradually increasing toward high, blend the ingredients for 30 to 45 seconds or until the mixture contains no visible pieces of fruit.
½ teaspoon ground cinnamon	
2 tablespoons raw cacao powder	
1 tablespoon maca powder	*3* Add the spinach and blend again at medium speed for 30 seconds, gradually increasing the speed to high. Blend on high speed for another 15 to 30 seconds or until the entire mixture is smooth.
2 Medjool dates, pitted	
6 raw unsalted cashews	
½-inch piece fresh ginger (peeled)	
2 cups water	*4* Pour the smoothie into two glasses and enjoy!
2 cups baby spinach, loosely packed	

Per serving: Calories 249 (From Fat 27); Fat 3g (Saturated 1g); Cholesterol 0mg; Sodium 40mg; Carbohydrate 54g (Dietary Fiber 8g); Protein 6g.

Tip: If you don't have fresh ginger, use ¼ teaspoon of ground ginger instead.

Vary It! If you want a spicy kick, add a dash of cayenne pepper instead of cinnamon. Instead of cashews, use 6 raw almonds or 2 tablespoons of cashew butter, almond butter, or tahini. Instead of Medjool dates, use 2 tablespoons of raw honey.

Pineapple Mango Coco-Yum

Prep time: 25 min • **Blending time:** 2 min • **Yield:** 2 servings

Ingredients	Directions
3 tablespoons goji berries	**1** Place the goji berries in a bowl with ¼ cup of room temperature water. Place in the fridge to soak for at least 20 minutes or overnight.
1 ripe mango	
1 cup pineapple chunks	
1 tablespoon bee pollen (omit if allergic)	**2** Peel the mango and cut the flesh away from the stone.
3 tablespoons coconut oil	
3 tablespoons shredded unsweetened coconut flakes	**3** Combine the goji berries, mango, pineapple, bee pollen, coconut oil, coconut flakes, and coconut water in the blender and secure the lid.
1½ cups coconut water	
½ cup arugula, loosely packed	
½ cup parsley, loosely packed	**4** Starting at low speed and gradually increasing toward high, blend the ingredients for 1 minute or until smooth.
¼ cup celery leaves, loosely packed	
	5 Add the arugula, parsley, and celery leaves (see Figure 9-2) and blend again at medium speed for 45 seconds, gradually increasing the speed to high.
	6 Pour the smoothie into two glasses, and enjoy!

Per serving: Calories 463 (From Fat 243); Fat 27g (Saturated 23g); Cholesterol 0mg; Sodium 223mg; Carbohydrate 53g (Dietary Fiber 8g); Protein 5g.

Tip: Arugula has a naturally spicy or peppery taste. Taste a leaf before adding it to your smoothie. If you don't like it, use 1 cup of spinach instead. And if you don't have mango, use 1 cup of fresh strawberries, raspberries, or blueberries.

Tip: For a fun presentation, serve this smoothie with a few coconut flakes on top.

Vary It! Add 1 ripe banana or ½ avocado to make the smoothie creamier.

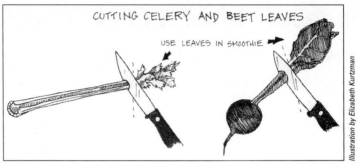

Figure 9-2: To use celery or beet greens, cut away the top leafy portion and set aside the main celery stalks or beets.

Illustration by Elizabeth Kurtzman

Soaking up benefits of soaked nuts and seeds

Ideally, you should soak nuts and seeds overnight before adding them to your smoothies because doing so removes the enzyme inhibitors and makes the food easier to digest. (*Enzyme inhibitors* are a natural coating on every nut and seed that keeps it from sprouting. Eating food with enzyme inhibitors can actually slow down or decrease your ability to fully digest food.) Some nuts taste better after soaking because they lose any bitterness. They usually blend better, too.

Remember: Be sure to rinse the nuts or seeds and drain the water that you soaked them in. Don't use the soaking water in your smoothie because that water contains the enzyme inhibitors that came off the nuts or seeds.

That said, anything good you're doing now is better than the bad you were doing before! If you're not ready to start soaking nuts yet, that's okay! Just toss them in dried or use raw nut butter instead. Find your own path and pace for making changes and that's your road to success.

Chapter 10

Evening Green Smoothies

. . . .

In This Chapter

▶ Preparing smoothies for fast and easy dinner options

▶ Making healthy evening desserts the family will love

. . . .

Did you ever even think of having a green smoothie for dinner? Or better yet, as a sweet and yummy dessert at the end of the day? Probably not, but in this chapter, I share five great recipes that will change the way you look at your evening meal and dessert.

If you find yourself always looking for something sweet to nibble on in the evening, you should try the sweet evening smoothie recipes in this chapter. They feed your sweet tooth without feeding your waistline. A healthy sweet smoothie gives your body added nutrients, fiber, alkalinity, chlorophyll, and healing power — the perfect way to end the day!

Considering the Sense of an Evening Smoothie

Perhaps you never thought to make a green smoothie in the evening, but sometimes that timing makes sense. Evening smoothies are a good idea if you fall into one of the following categories:

✔ You have one really busy night a week when you usually order takeout and are ready to change to something healthy instead.

✔ You have limited time in the evening because of night classes or a late shift and you want to make something healthy but fast to get you back out the door in a jiffy.

✔ You want to go to the gym or work out at night but don't want to eat a heavy meal beforehand.

Saving time by presoaking chia seeds

I recommend you always have some chia seeds soaking in the fridge, ready to add to a green smoothie anytime. That way, you don't have to wait around for 20 minutes when you want to blend up a smoothie now. The seeds remain fresh in the fridge for three to four days while soaking. Soak 4 to 6 tablespoons at a time in a glass container with a sealed lid.

✔ You ate too much over the weekend and want to have a light dinner to make up for it.

✔ You tend to be a late-night snacker and are looking for better options as a transition to stop snacking once and for all.

✔ You and your family enjoy having dessert but want to upgrade to a healthy version of something sweet.

Keep your goals in mind as you read through the recipes in this chapter. You may just find the perfect smoothie to fit your evening needs!

Double-checking essential oils

Many products claiming to be essential oils aren't pure extracts and often contain fillers and even added chemicals. You definitely shouldn't use those oils in recipes! Check the labels of your essential oils; they should read "100% Pure Essential Oil," "Therapeutic Grade," or both.

South of the Border Spicy

Prep time: 4–5 min • **Blending time:** 2 min • **Yield:** 2 servings

Ingredients	Directions
½ avocado, peeled and pitted 2 ripe tomatoes, halved 1 cup peeled, chopped cucumber 2 tablespoons fresh lime juice Pinch of cayenne pepper to taste 1 cup water ½ cup cilantro, loosely packed 1½ cups baby spinach, loosely packed ¼ teaspoon chopped fresh jalapeño pepper, seeded (optional)	*1* Combine the avocado, tomatoes, cucumber, lime juice, cayenne, and water in the blender and secure the lid. *2* Starting at low speed and gradually increasing toward high, blend the ingredients for 30 to 45 seconds or until the mixture contains no visible pieces of fruit. *3* Add the cilantro and spinach and blend again at medium speed for 30 seconds, gradually increasing the speed to high. Blend on high speed for another 15 to 30 seconds or until the entire mixture is smooth. *4* Turn the blender off and taste the smoothie. If you want it spicier, add the jalapeño and blend again for 15 seconds or until smooth. *5* Pour the smoothie into two glasses and enjoy!

Per serving: Calories 96 (From Fat 54); Fat 6g (Saturated 1g); Cholesterol 0mg; Sodium 32mg; Carbohydrate 11g (Dietary Fiber 5g); Protein 3g.

Tip: You can pour this smoothie into bowls and eat it with a spoon, like a soup.

Tip: Add a pinch of Himalayan salt to bring out more of the savory flavors. Look for this salt in health food stores or online.

Vary It! If you like fresh garlic, try adding a peeled clove with the ingredients in Step 1. You can also add ½ cup of fresh celery leaves in Step 3 for even more greens.

Green Gazpacho with Sprouts

Prep time: 4–5 min • **Blending time:** 3 min • **Yield:** 2 servings

Ingredients	Directions
1 red or yellow bell pepper 3 medium cucumbers	**1** Cut the bell pepper into quarters and remove the seeds. Peel and chop the cucumbers.
¼ cup mung bean sprouts 1 garlic clove, peeled ¼ cup fresh lime juice	**2** Combine the bell pepper, cucumber, mung beans, garlic, lime juice, vinegar, cayenne, and salt in the blender and secure the lid.
1 tablespoon raw apple cider vinegar Pinch of cayenne pepper to taste	**3** Starting at low speed and gradually increasing toward high, blend the ingredients for 30 to 45 seconds or until smooth.
Himalayan salt to taste 1½ cups spinach, loosely packed ¼ cup alfalfa, lentil, or radish sprouts	**4** Add the spinach and blend again at medium speed for 30 seconds, gradually increasing the speed to high. Blend on high speed for another 15 to 30 seconds or until the entire mixture is smooth.
	5 Pour the smoothie into two bowls. Garnish with the alfalfa, lentil, or radish sprouts. Enjoy!

Per serving: Calories 67 (From Fat 5); Fat 0.5g (Saturated 0g); Cholesterol 0mg; Sodium 167mg; Carbohydrate 0g (Dietary Fiber 3g); Protein 3g.

Tip: If the smoothie tastes too bland, add extra Himalayan salt or cayenne pepper and blend again for 15 seconds or until smooth.

Shaping your smoothie routine

The most important factor in knowing when to drink your smoothie is to find the best time that works for you. Your body absorbs all the nutrients whether your smoothie is your breakfast, nighttime snack, or something in between. And you don't have to commit to the same timing every day. Monday night may be your crazy busy evening, so maybe that's the night to have a smoothie for dinner. The rest of the weekdays, your schedule may dictate that having a smoothie for breakfast is best; on the weekends, you may enjoy having a green smoothie in the early afternoon. Experiment with having smoothies for breakfast, lunch, or dinner and see what works best for you. Any combination is okay!

Cool Mint Chocolate Chip

Prep time: 3 min • **Blending time:** 2 min • **Yield:** 2 servings

Ingredients	Directions
1 red apple	*1* Cut the apple and remove the core, keeping the skin intact. Cut the flesh into quarters.
2 ripe bananas, peeled	
1 tablespoon raw honey	
2 tablespoons ground flaxseed	*2* Combine the apple, banana, honey, flaxseed, cacao powder, peppermint oil, and water in the blender and secure the lid.
1½ tablespoons raw cacao powder	
1–2 drops pure peppermint essential oil	*3* Starting at low speed and gradually increasing toward high, blend the ingredients for 30 to 45 seconds or until the mixture contains no visible pieces of fruit.
1½ cups water	
1½ cups chopped bok choy, loosely packed	*4* Add the bok choy and blend again at medium speed for 30 seconds, gradually increasing the speed to high. Blend on high speed for another 30 seconds or until the entire mixture is smooth.
1 tablespoon raw cacao nibs	
2–3 mint leaves	
	5 Add the cacao nibs and blend again for just 5 to 10 seconds.
	6 Pour the smoothie into two glasses. Garnish with the fresh mint leaves. Enjoy!

Per serving: Calories 291 (From Fat 63); Fat 7g (Saturated 2.5g); Cholesterol 0mg; Sodium 47mg; Carbohydrate 56g (Dietary Fiber 10g); Protein 5g.

Tip: If the smoothie is too thick, add ½ cup of additional water after Step 5 and blend again. To boost the chocolate chip taste, add an additional tablespoon of raw cacao nibs in Step 5.

Vary It! Try carob powder instead of raw cacao powder. For an orange-chocolate smoothie taste, add 1 or 2 drops of wild orange essential oil instead of peppermint oil. If the bok choy is too spicy or bitter for your taste, replace it with 1½ cups of fresh spinach.

Vary It! You can also add frozen banana to get more of an ice cream texture. In that case, peel the ripe bananas, cut them into chunks, and place the chopped banana in a plastic bag in the freezer. Allow it to freeze overnight, and add it to your smoothie the next day.

Sweet Vanilla Cacao Dessert

Prep time: 4–5 min • **Blending time:** 2 min • **Yield:** 2 servings

Ingredients	*Directions*
½ avocado, peeled and pitted 2 Medjool dates, pitted 1 ripe banana, peeled 8 raw Brazil nuts 2 tablespoons raw cacao powder 1 tablespoon raw cacao butter 2 teaspoons vanilla extract 1 cup water 1½ cups spinach, loosely packed	*1* Combine the avocado, dates, banana, Brazil nuts, cacao powder, cacao butter, vanilla, and water in the blender and secure the lid. *2* Starting at low speed and gradually increasing toward high, blend the ingredients for 30 to 45 seconds or until the mixture contains no visible pieces of fruit. *3* Add the spinach and blend again at medium speed for 30 seconds, gradually increasing the speed to high. Blend on high speed for another 15 to 30 seconds or until the entire mixture is smooth.
1 tablespoon raw cacao nibs	*4* Add the cacao nibs and blend again for just 5 to 10 seconds. Pour the smoothie into two glasses and enjoy!

Per serving: Calories 355 (From Fat 180); Fat 20g (Saturated 8g); Cholesterol 0mg; Sodium 28mg; Carbohydrate 42g (Dietary Fiber 9g); Protein 5g.

Tip: As a nice garnish, serve this smoothie with a sprinkle of raw cacao nibs on top.

Tip: If you don't have Brazil nuts, use 10 to 12 raw cashews instead. If you don't have cacao butter, use 1 tablespoon of coconut oil.

Tip: If the smoothie tastes bitter to you, try sweetening it up by adding 1 tablespoon of raw honey, or a second Medjool date, or ½ teaspoon of stevia powder.

Cacao powder, nibs, *and* butter?

Is it really necessary to add three different cacao ingredients in one smoothie? Well, yes and no. *Cacao powder* adds that pure raw chocolate taste. *Cacao nibs* are little chips or pieces of cacao, and they add a chocolate-chip-like texture. *Cacao butter* is smooth and creamy and adds a very sweet taste and creamy texture. If you only use cacao powder, your smoothie will still taste great. Adding all three cacao ingredients just gives more subtle levels of extra taste.

Blue Green Dream

Prep time: 25 min • **Blending time:** 2 min • **Yield:** 2 servings

Ingredients	Directions
2 tablespoons chia seeds	*1* Place the chia seeds in a bowl with ¼ cup of room temperature water. Place in the fridge to soak for at least 20 minutes or overnight.
2 red apples	
1 cup blueberries	
¼ cup fresh lemon juice	*2* Cut the apples and remove the core, keeping the skin intact. Cut the flesh into quarters.
1½ cups water	
½ cup parsley, loosely packed	*3* Combine the apples, blueberries, chia seeds with soaking water, lemon juice, and water in the blender and secure the lid.
1½ cups watercress, loosely packed	
3–4 mint leaves	*4* Starting at low speed and gradually increasing toward high, blend the ingredients for 30 to 45 seconds or until the mixture contains no visible pieces of fruit.
	5 Add the parsley, watercress, and mint leaves and blend again at medium speed for 30 seconds, gradually increasing the speed to high. Blend on high speed for another 30 seconds or until the entire mixture is smooth.
	6 Pour the smoothie into two glasses and enjoy!

Per serving: Calories 224 (From Fat 45); Fat 5g (Saturated 0.5g); Cholesterol 0mg; Sodium 30mg; Carbohydrate 45g (Dietary Fiber 12g); Protein 5g.

Tip: If you don't like the taste of mint, you can leave it out. Just add a few more leaves of fresh parsley instead. And if fresh berries aren't in season, substitute them with 1 tablespoon of acai powder or 1 tablespoon of pomegranate powder.

Vary It! For a creamier texture, add 1 ripe banana or ¼ avocado. Try fresh raspberries or strawberries instead of blueberries.

Chapter 11

Green Smoothies for Kids

Starting your children with healthy food and eating patterns at the earliest age possible gives them a foundation of good healthy habits for life. Make healthy eating fun and adventurous by introducing new foods and creating new recipes with different ingredients. As you bring new fruits or greens into your home, explain to your kids why each food is good for them. When you see them choosing healthy foods, praise them for their good choices.

This chapter presents green smoothie recipes for kids at every age, from baby to toddler to adolescent. If your family is new to green smoothies, start slowly. Use half the leafy greens listed in each recipe, replacing them with more fruits until the kids get used to the taste. Gradually, you can increase to the full amount of greens.

Perfect Transition! Making Green Smoothies Baby's First Food

Somewhere between the ages of 7 and 9 months, your baby will be ready to make the transition to solid food. (The exact age varies depending on whether your baby is bottle- or breast-fed.) An easy-to-digest blended green smoothie is the perfect choice for a healthy transitional food from formula or milk to solid foods.

The benefits of giving your baby green smoothies include the following:

- ✔ They're easy to digest in a blended form.
- ✔ They offer valuable nutrients from the fruits and leafy greens.
- ✔ They help relieve constipation, a condition that often occurs as babies transition to solid foods.
- ✔ They're more affordable than store-bought baby food.
- ✔ They're fresher and more natural than canned baby food (no added refined sugar or preservatives).

Whether you're bottle- or breast-feeding, you can give your baby a small amount of green smoothie in a sippy cup once or twice a day before feeding, and then finish off with the bottle or breast milk. You can store any leftovers in the fridge for up to 24 hours, which helps save time for subsequent feedings later in the day.

Depending on the size of your baby's sippy cup straw, you may have to dilute the smoothie with an additional ½ to 1 cup of water in each recipe.

Good first fruits for babies are usually banana, pear, apple, mango, avocado, or peach. Good leafy greens for babies include kale and spinach. Some babies do react to strawberries, raspberries, or blackberries, so avoid those when first introducing new foods. Blueberries, however, are usually okay.

Before you start giving your baby any of these recipes, offer a single food ingredient first (such as peaches or avocado) and wait for three to four days. During that time, watch for any signs of allergy such as diarrhea, vomiting, rash, or wheezing. If your baby tolerates the food well, you can use it in the smoothie recipe. Here are some other tips for baby smoothies:

- ✔ Blend the smoothie completely; check that no small bits are remaining.
- ✔ Choose organic produce and wash it well (see Chapter 3).
- ✔ Alternate greens for each smoothie. For example, use baby spinach one day and baby kale the next.
- ✔ In the beginning, feed your baby green smoothies every other day until his or her digestive tract gets used to them.
- ✔ Add healthy fats, such as avocado or small amounts of coconut or flaxseed oil.

Pear and Spinach Baby Green Smile

Prep time: 2 min • **Blending time:** 1 min • **Yield:** 2 servings

Ingredients	Directions
1 ripe pear	**1** Cut the pear and remove the core, keeping the skin intact. Cut the flesh into quarters.
1 ripe banana, peeled	
1 cup water	**2** Combine the pear, banana, and water in the blender and secure the lid.
1 cup baby spinach, loosely packed	
	3 Starting at low speed and gradually increasing toward high, blend the ingredients for 15 to 20 seconds or until the mixture contains no visible pieces of fruit.
	4 Add the spinach and blend again at medium speed for 15 to 30 seconds, gradually increasing the speed to high. Blend on high speed for another 10 seconds or until the entire mixture is smooth.
	5 Pour half the smoothie into a bowl or sippy cup and serve. Drink the remaining smoothie yourself or refrigerate it in a sealed container for up to 24 hours.

Per serving: Calories 103 (From Fat 4); Fat 0.5g (Saturated 0g); Cholesterol 0mg; Sodium 16mg; Carbohydrate 27g (Dietary Fiber 4g); Protein 1g.

Vary It! Try adding 1 ripe peach instead of pear.

Taking care with superfood powders in smoothies for babies

Some parents ask whether adding spirulina or other superfood powders to a baby's diet is okay. I advise you to avoid these ingredients until you see how well your child is digesting and assimilating food. If everything that goes in is coming out in a healthy, formed, and consistent manner, you can start adding ¼ teaspoon of spirulina powder to any of the baby or toddler recipes. Avoid using chlorella powder due to high risk of allergic reaction. Use whole fruits or berries instead of superfood berry powders. Whole foods with the fiber are the best foods for a growing child.

Apple, Avocado, and Baby Kale Love

Prep time: 2 min • **Blending time:** 1 min • **Yield:** 2 servings

Ingredients	Directions
1 red delicious or gala apple	*1* Cut the apple and remove the core, keeping the skin intact. Cut the flesh into quarters.
½ avocado, peeled and pitted	
1 cup water	*2* Combine the apple, avocado, and water in the blender and secure the lid.
2 baby kale leaves	
	3 Starting at low speed and gradually increasing toward high, blend the ingredients for 15 to 20 seconds or until the mixture contains no visible pieces of fruit.
	4 Add the kale and blend again at medium speed for 15 to 30 seconds, gradually increasing the speed to high. Blend on high speed for another 10 seconds or until the entire mixture is smooth.
	5 Pour half the smoothie into a bowl or sippy cup and serve. Drink the remaining smoothie yourself or refrigerate it in a sealed container for up to 24 hours.

Per serving: Calories 120 (From Fat 54); Fat 6g (Saturated 1g); Cholesterol 0mg; Sodium 20mg; Carbohydrate 18g (Dietary Fiber 5g); Protein 2g.

Tip: If you can't find baby kale, use 1 cup of baby spinach instead.

Mango and Peach Sunshine

Prep time: 2 min • **Blending time:** 2 min • **Yield:** 2 servings

Ingredients	Directions
1 ripe mango **1 ripe peach** **1½ cups water** **1 cup baby spinach, loosely packed**	*1* Peel the mango and cut the flesh away from the stone. Cut the peach and remove the stone, keeping the skin intact. Cut the flesh of both fruits into quarters.
	2 Combine the mango, peach, and water in the blender and secure the lid.
	3 Starting at low speed and gradually increasing toward high, blend the ingredients for 15 to 30 seconds or until smooth.
	4 Add the spinach and blend again at medium speed for 30 to 45 seconds, gradually increasing the speed to high.
	5 Pour half the smoothie into a bowl or sippy cup and serve. Drink the remaining smoothie yourself or refrigerate it in a sealed container for up to 24 hours.

Per serving: *Calories 97 (From Fat 4); Fat 0.5g (Saturated 0g); Cholesterol 0mg; Sodium 27mg; Carbohydrate 24g (Dietary Fiber 3g); Protein 2g.*

K.I.S.S.: Keep it sweet and simple

Remember the basic K.I.S.S. rule as you experiment with new green smoothie recipes for your baby or toddler: Keep it sweet and simple. Babies like the sweet taste of fruits such as banana or apple, so always include something that's naturally sweet. Then keep the rest of the recipe simple. Limit the number of additional ingredients to just three or four, making an easy-to-digest smoothie for a baby's tummy.

Banana and Prune Paradise

Prep time: 2–3 min • **Blending time:** 1 min • **Yield:** 2 servings

Ingredients	Directions
1 ripe banana, peeled	*1* Combine the banana, prunes, coconut oil, and water in the blender and secure the lid.
2 pitted prunes	
1 teaspoon coconut oil	*2* Starting at low speed and gradually increasing toward high, blend the ingredients for 15 to 30 seconds or until the mixture contains no visible pieces of fruit.
1½ cups water	
2 romaine lettuce leaves	
	3 Add the romaine and blend again at medium speed for 30 seconds, gradually increasing the speed to high. Blend on high speed for another 15 to 30 seconds or until the entire mixture is smooth.
	4 Pour half the smoothie into a bowl or sippy cup and serve. Drink the remaining smoothie yourself or refrigerate it in a sealed container for up to 24 hours.

Per serving: Calories 130 (From Fat 23); Fat 2.5g (Saturated 2g); Cholesterol 0mg; Sodium 7mg; Carbohydrate 27g (Dietary Fiber 2g); Protein 1g.

Make it a family habit and a family meal

A lot of kids are picky eaters, and out of desperation, many parents make separate meals for their kids in the hopes that the children will just eat *something*. As a result, the dinner table gets divided between adult food and kid food. Using that approach can have long-term consequences and make getting children to eat their vegetables, or any healthy food, even harder. After kids identify a difference between adult and kid foods, they think that they can eat according to their preference, and they won't want to give up that luxury so easily!

Every time you make green smoothies, make enough for the whole family and serve everyone a glass. Allow your child to watch each family member eating the same food from the earliest age possible. Children will copy what they see even if they're too young to know exactly what's happening. As your baby transitions to solid food, uphold the one meal per family rule. Always have at least one food on your plate that your baby is eating too, such as mashed sweet potato or pureed soup.

Heavenly Papaya and Coconut Water

Prep time: 3–4 min • **Blending time:** 2 min • **Yield:** 2 servings

Ingredients	Directions
1 ripe banana, peeled	*1* Combine the banana, papaya, and coconut water in the blender and secure the lid.
1 cup ripe chopped papaya (peeled and seeded)	
1 cup coconut water	*2* Starting at low speed and gradually increasing toward high, blend the ingredients for 15 to 30 seconds or until the mixture contains no visible pieces of fruit.
2 baby kale leaves	
	3 Add the kale and blend again at medium speed for 15 to 30 seconds, gradually increasing the speed to high. Blend on high speed for another 10 seconds or until the entire mixture is smooth.
	4 Pour half the smoothie into a bowl or sippy cup and serve. Drink the remaining smoothie yourself or refrigerate in a sealed container for up to 24 hours.

Per serving: Calories 122 (From Fat 9); Fat 1g (Saturated 0.5g); Cholesterol 0mg; Sodium 145mg; Carbohydrate 28g (Dietary Fiber 5g); Protein 3g.

Tip: If you don't have fresh papaya, use 1 cup of fresh pineapple instead. If you can't find baby kale, use 1 cup of baby spinach instead.

Trying Toddlers' Green Smoothies

Between 12 and 36 months of age, your child begins self-feeding and may show more eagerness in making food choices. Take advantage of her interest by offering different colors of smoothie cups or giving her a choice between banana and avocado for her green smoothie.

At the toddler age, your child is acutely aware of everything you do, so be a good role model. Pour a cup of green smoothie for your little one and a large glass for you and drink it together.

Leafy greens contain calcium, iron, and vitamin C, all fantastic nutrients for a growing toddler. Green smoothies are a great medium for adding supplements to your toddler's diet. The top smoothie ingredients to use for toddlers are

- **Blackstrap molasses:** Provides a good plant-based source of iron

- **Raw honey:** Boosts immune system and reduces risk of seasonal allergies

- **Carob powder:** Promotes regular bowel movements and helps stabilize blood sugars

- **Ground flaxseed:** Offers a great source of fiber and omega-3 fatty acids

- **Flaxseed oil:** Strengthens digestion and provides omega-3 fatty acids

- **Chia seeds:** Add protein, fiber, and omega-3 fatty acids

Experiment with different combinations, but don't use more than one new supplement at a time, and monitor your child for any reactions. In addition, you can add a probiotic capsule in Step 2 of any recipe before blending for good gut bacteria, especially after a course of antibiotics.

Doctors recommend that you wait until your child is at least 1 year old to give her honey or bee products, and then, introduce them slowly. First, feed her a small amount (about ½ teaspoon) and wait two to three days. If she doesn't experience swelling, rashes, or noticeable discomfort, gradually increase the serving to 1 tablespoon (stopping if you notice any side effects at one of the intermediate doses).

Orange, Carob, and Almond Milk Serenade

Prep time: 3–4 min • **Blending time:** 2 min • **Yield:** 2 servings

Ingredients	Directions
1 orange, peeled and seeded ½ cup raspberries ½ teaspoon carob powder ½ cup water 1 cup homemade almond milk 1 cup baby spinach, loosely packed	**1** Combine the orange, raspberries, carob powder, water, and almond milk in the blender and secure the lid. **2** Starting at low speed and gradually increasing toward high, blend the ingredients for 30 to 45 seconds or until the mixture contains no visible pieces of fruit. **3** Add the spinach and blend again at medium speed for 15 to 20 seconds, gradually increasing the speed to high. Blend on high speed for another 15 seconds or until the entire mixture is smooth. **4** Pour the smoothie into two cups and enjoy!

Per serving: Calories 71 (From Fat 18); Fat 2g (Saturated 0g); Cholesterol 0mg; Sodium 103mg; Carbohydrate 13g (Dietary Fiber 5g); Protein 2g.

Tip: Chapter 6 has instructions on making almond milk. If you don't have homemade almond milk, add ¼ cup of raw almonds and 1 cup of additional water instead in Step 1.

Tip: If your child is sensitive to raspberries, add 1 peeled ripe banana instead.

Blueberry, Molasses, and Apple Supreme

Prep time: 3–4 min • **Blending time:** 2 min • **Yield:** 2 servings

Ingredients	Directions
1 red delicious or gala apple ½ cup blueberries	*1* Cut the apple and remove the core, keeping the skin intact. Cut the flesh into quarters.
1 ripe banana, peeled 1 tablespoon blackstrap molasses	*2* Combine the apple, blueberries, banana, molasses, and water in the blender and secure the lid.
1½ cups water 2 Swiss chard leaves	*3* Starting at low speed and gradually increasing toward high, blend the ingredients for 30 to 45 seconds or until the mixture contains no visible pieces of fruit.
	4 Remove and discard the Swiss chard stems. Roughly chop or tear the leaves, add them to the blender, and blend again at medium speed for 15 to 20 seconds, gradually increasing the speed to high. Blend on high speed for another 15 seconds or until the entire mixture is smooth.
	5 Pour the smoothie into two cups and enjoy!

Per serving: Calories 146 (From Fat 4); Fat 0.5g (Saturated 0g); Cholesterol 0mg; Sodium 41mg; Carbohydrate 38g (Dietary Fiber 5g); Protein 1g.

Tip: Add a dash of ground cinnamon for a slightly sweet taste.

Amazing Grape, Honey, and Pear

Prep time: 3–4 min • **Blending time:** 2 min • **Yield:** 2 servings

Ingredients	Directions
1 ripe pear **½ avocado, peeled and pitted** **1 cup red or green grapes** **1 tablespoon raw honey** **1½ cups water** **1 cup baby bok choy leaves, loosely packed**	*1* Cut the pear and remove the core, keeping the skin intact. Cut the flesh into quarters. Combine the pear, avocado, grapes, honey, and water in the blender and secure the lid. *2* Starting at low speed and gradually increasing toward high, blend the ingredients for 30 to 45 seconds or until the mixture contains no visible pieces of fruit. *3* Add the bok choy and blend again at medium speed for 15 to 20 seconds, gradually increasing the speed to high. Blend on high speed for another 15 seconds or until the entire mixture is smooth. *4* Pour the smoothie into two cups and enjoy!

Per serving: *Calories 192 (From Fat 45); Fat 5g (Saturated 1g); Cholesterol 0mg; Sodium 34mg; Carbohydrate 39g (Dietary Fiber 6g); Protein 2g.*

Vary It! Instead of grapes, add 1 cup of frozen organic cherries.

Making smoothies fun for kids

Here are some additional kid-friendly tips for green smoothies:

- Let your child help pick out fruits in the store.
- Name your green-colored smoothie after a favorite green character.
- Add appealing garnishes, such as a slice of banana or strawberry with a sprinkle of unsweetened coconut flakes.
- Freeze smoothies into silicone molds with wooden sticks and serve as green smoothie popsicles.
- Set a routine and boundaries for healthy eating. If you see that your child didn't drink any smoothie but asks for a not-so-healthy snack later, be prepared and stay consistent with your answer. Try something like "Did you finish your smoothie today? I give treats to kids who finish their healthy green drink. Are you ready to drink some green smoothie? I'll pour some for myself, too."

Apricot and Strawberries Forever Young

Prep time: 3–4 min • **Blending time:** 2 min • **Yield:** 2 servings

Ingredients	Directions
2 ripe apricots **1 ripe banana, peeled** **½ cup halved strawberries, stems and leaves removed** **1 teaspoon ground flaxseed** **1 teaspoon flaxseed oil** **1½ cups water** **3 baby kale leaves**	**1** Cut the apricots and remove the stones, keeping the skin intact. Cut the flesh into quarters. **2** Combine all the ingredients except the kale in the blender and secure the lid. **3** Starting at low speed and gradually increasing toward high, blend the ingredients for 30 to 45 seconds or the mixture contains no visible pieces of fruit. **4** Add the kale and blend again at medium speed for 15 to 20 seconds, gradually increasing the speed to high. Blend on high speed for another 15 seconds or until the entire mixture is smooth. **5** Pour the smoothie into two cups and enjoy!

Per serving: Calories 123 (From Fat 36); Fat 4g (Saturated 0.5g); Cholesterol 0g; Sodium 20mg; Carbohydrate 23g (Dietary Fiber 4g); Protein 3g.

Tip: If your child is sensitive to strawberries, add ½ cup of fresh blueberries instead. If you can't find baby kale, use 1 cup of baby spinach instead.

Vary It! Use 4 dried organic apricots (soaked in water for 20 minutes) or 1 fresh peach (skin on and stone removed) in place of the ripe apricots.

Using baby leaves for babies and toddlers

It's no coincidence that nearly all the baby and toddler green smoothie recipes in this chapter include baby leaves, such as baby kale, baby spinach, or baby bok choy. The baby leaves are often milder in taste, making them a more suitable choice for a small child's palate. Other options for mild greens include celery leaves, Swiss chard, or romaine lettuce.

Melon and Mint Refresher

Prep time: 25 min • **Blending time:** 2 min • **Yield:** 2 servings

Ingredients	Directions
1 tablespoon chia seeds 1½ cups chopped cantaloupe 1 cup water 3 fresh mint leaves ½ cup baby spinach, loosely packed	**1** Place the chia seeds in a bowl with ¼ cup of room temperature water. Place in the fridge to soak for at least 20 minutes or overnight. **2** Combine the chia seeds, cantaloupe, and water in the blender and secure the lid. **3** Starting at low speed and gradually increasing toward high, blend the ingredients for 30 to 45 seconds or until the mixture contains no visible pieces of fruit. **4** Add the mint and spinach and blend again at a medium speed for 15 to 20 seconds, gradually increasing the speed to high. Blend on high speed for another 15 seconds or until the entire mixture is smooth. **5** Pour the smoothie into two cups and enjoy!

Per serving: Calories 79 (From Fat 23); Fat 2.5g (Saturated 0.5g); Cholesterol 0mg; Sodium 29mg; Carbohydrate 13g (Dietary Fiber 4g); Protein 2g.

Vary It! Add a peeled banana for a creamier texture and taste.

Healthy is Cool! Gearing Green Smoothies toward Teens

Even if you didn't start your children on green smoothies at an early age, there's definitely hope for them in their older years. As your kids get older, take the time to emphasize the importance of healthy foods for their mental performance at school, their physical performance with sports, and their highest chances of succeeding as adults. After all, if you're tired and don't feel good, can you really expect to ace your tests, stay energized during the game, and impress recruiters in getting a job? These are just some of the reasons to get a daily green smoothie in your teenager's diet. And remember, you're your child's best role model, so you need to drink green smoothies too!

Green smoothies are great for teens for several reasons:

- ✔ They clear your skin and minimize breakouts.

- ✔ They give you shiny, thick, healthy hair.

- ✔ They give your eyes a bright sparkle.

- ✔ They keep your teeth white and reduce tooth decay.

- ✔ They boost your energy.

- ✔ They help you concentrate better at school.

- ✔ They build muscle and improve endurance, which is particularly good for sports.

- ✔ They strengthen your immune system.

- ✔ They help regulate weight (thanks to the fiber).

As your kids get older, let them make their own smoothies and encourage them to try new combinations. Offer them to use healthy superfoods such as raw cacao powder, carob powder, spirulina powder, hemp powder, or coconut oil. Even ingredients like peanut butter or yogurt are okay if using them means your teenager is actually drinking a green smoothie. Remember, a green smoothie with dairy or peanut butter is better than no green smoothie at all! You may be surprised to see what new recipes they create!

Check out www.dummies.com/extras/greensmoothies for a Tahini and Coconut Anytime Snack green smoothie recipe.

Pineapple and Grape Pick-Me-Up

Prep time: 3–4 min • **Blending time:** 2 min • **Yield:** 2 servings

Ingredients	Directions
1 cup pineapple chunks	**1** Combine all the ingredients except the spinach in the blender and secure the lid.
1 ripe banana, peeled	
1 cup red or green grapes	**2** Starting at low speed and gradually increasing toward high, blend the ingredients for 30 to 45 seconds or until the mixture contains no visible pieces of fruit.
2 tablespoons ground flaxseed	
1 teaspoon spirulina powder	
1½ cups water	
2 cups baby spinach leaves, loosely packed	**3** Add the spinach and blend again at medium speed for 30 to 45 seconds, gradually increasing the speed to high. Blend on high speed for another 15 to 20 seconds or until the entire mixture is smooth. Pour the smoothie into two glasses and enjoy!

Per serving: Calories 215 (From Fat 23); Fat 2.5g (Saturated 0g); Cholesterol 0mg; Sodium 56mg; Carbohydrate 47g (Dietary Fiber 6g); Protein 4g.

Tip: Pack one serving in a plastic container and place in a cooler with an ice pack. Send it to school with your teen for a mid-morning or afternoon snack.

Making smoothies for the entire family

How do you make green smoothies for yourself, your spouse, and kids of various ages all at once? Make your smoothies in stages, adding more ingredients with each step. Here's how it works:

1. Start with the simplest recipe first. For example, if you have a baby or toddler, make her smoothie with just a few simple ingredients and pour it into a sippy cup.

2. Add some flaxseed, spirulina, honey, dates, another banana, or berries to the remaining ingredients in the blender and blend again. Add more greens and blend until smooth. Pour into a glass and hand off to the teenager running by.

3. Make the last batch of smoothies for the adults. Add your ingredients with water and blend. You don't even have to clean the blender in between.

In less than 10 minutes, everyone's got a green smoothie in hand, and your entire family is making a healthy start to the day.

Apple and Lime Bright-Eyed Morning Tang

Prep time: 3–4 min • **Blending time:** 2 min • **Yield:** 2 servings

Ingredients	Directions
2 red delicious or gala apples	*1* Cut the apples and remove the cores, keeping the skin intact. Cut the flesh into quarters. Combine all the ingredients except the celery leaves in the blender and secure the lid.
½ avocado, peeled and pitted	
Juice of ¼ lime	*2* Starting at low speed and gradually increasing toward high, blend the ingredients for 30 to 45 seconds or until the mixture contains no visible pieces of fruit.
2 tablespoons ground hemp seed	*3* Add the celery leaves and blend again at medium speed for 30 seconds, gradually increasing the speed to high. Blend on high speed for another 15 to 20 seconds or until the entire mixture is smooth.
1½ cups water	
1 cup celery leaves, loosely packed	*4* Pour the smoothie into two glasses and enjoy!

Per serving: Calories 244 (From Fat 117); Fat 13g (Saturated 1g); Cholesterol 0mg; Sodium 50mg; Carbohydrate 32g (Dietary Fiber 9g); Protein 7g.

Taking the edge off teenager moodiness

Hormonal changes are at least partly to blame for your adolescent's mood swings and unpredictable bouts of irritability. But the food that teens eat can really affect them, too. Emotions can get more intense if your teenager is fatigued or eating poorly. Having a good foundation of healthy eating habits is the key to minimizing mood swings and creating a more peaceful household for your entire family. Of course, a few door-slamming and feet-stomping episodes are still bound to occur, but they'll be greatly reduced with a balanced diet high in fresh fruits and veggies. Here are some ways to thwart the diet-related outbursts:

✔ Ensure everyone eats breakfast, lunch, and dinner (no meal skipping).

✔ Use green smoothies to increase your teen's green leafy vegetable intake (for iron and zinc) and fruit intake (for B vitamins).

✔ Keep caffeinated energy drinks and high-sugar snacks out of the pantry. In addition to green smoothies, have plenty of fresh fruits, nuts, and seeds on-hand as healthy alternatives.

Banana and Brazil Nut Brain Fuel

Prep time: 3–4 min • **Blending time:** 2 min • **Yield:** 2 servings

Ingredients	Directions
2 ripe bananas, peeled **1 cup halved strawberries, stems and leaves removed**	*1* Combine the bananas, strawberries, dates, Brazil nuts, and water in the blender and secure the lid.
2 Medjool dates, pitted **6 raw Brazil nuts** **2 cups water**	*2* Starting at low speed and gradually increasing toward high, blend the ingredients for 30 to 45 seconds or until the mixture contains no visible pieces of fruit.
¼ cup fresh parsley **2 large kale leaves**	*3* Remove and discard the kale stems. Add the kale and parsley and blend again at medium speed for 30 seconds, gradually increasing the speed to high. Blend on high speed for another 15 to 20 seconds or until the entire mixture is smooth.
	4 Pour the smoothie into two glasses and enjoy!

Per serving: Calories 323 (From Fat 108); Fat 12g (Saturated 2.5g); Cholesterol 0mg; Sodium 27mg; Carbohydrate 56g (Dietary Fiber 8g); Protein 6g.

Tip: If you don't have Brazil nuts, use 6 raw walnut halves instead.

Vary It! Instead of strawberries, try 1 fresh peach (skin on and stone removed).

After-School Peachy Berry and Orange

Prep time: 25 min • **Blending time:** 2 min • **Yield:** 2 servings

Ingredients	Directions
2 tablespoons chia seeds	**1** Place the chia seeds in a bowl with ¼ cup of room temperature water. Place in the fridge to soak for at least 20 minutes or overnight.
2 ripe peaches	
1 orange, peeled and seeded	
1 cup raspberries	**2** Cut the peaches and remove the stones, keeping the skin intact. Cut the flesh into quarters.
1 teaspoon spirulina powder	
1½ cups water	
3 mint leaves	**3** Combine the chia seeds, peaches, orange, raspberries, spirulina powder, and water in the blender and secure the lid.
4 large romaine lettuce leaves	
	4 Starting at low speed and gradually increasing toward high, blend the ingredients for 30 to 45 seconds or until smooth.
	5 Add the mint and romaine and blend again at medium speed for 15 to 30 seconds, gradually increasing the speed to high. Blend on high speed for another 15 to 20 seconds or until the entire mixture is smooth.
	6 Pour the smoothie into two glasses and enjoy!

Per serving: Calories 202 (From Fat 54); Fat 6g (Saturated 0.5g); Cholesterol 0mg; Sodium 27mg; Carbohydrate 37g (Dietary Fiber 13g); Protein 6g.

Vary It! Add 1 banana instead of 1 orange for a smoother, creamier texture. Add ¼ teaspoon of ground ginger for a warm and spicy flavor.

Part IV

Green Smoothies to Meet Your Individual Health Needs

Five Tips for Successful Weight Loss Smoothies

- **Good fats are good, but you can definitely have too many when trying to lose weight.** Cut back on the fat calories in a smoothie, and you won't even notice the difference. Save the avocado for later to enjoy in a salad and keep the nuts as a snack (one handful per day is best).

- **Cut out the coconut oil.** Coconut oil has a whopping 117 calories in just 1 tablespoon! Avoid using coconut oil in smoothies when your goal is weight loss. When you're back in maintenance mode or as you start to exercise more, you can add it back in.

- **Use bananas sparingly.** Banana is an excellent fruit and high in fiber, but also packs some calories. If you can't lose the banana altogether, use just half in a smoothie to spread your caloric load throughout the day.

- **Add more water.** Get the feeling of eating more and dilute the natural sugars in your smoothie by simply adding more water. During a weight loss regimen, you can use 2 to 3 cups instead of the normal 1½ cups of water per recipe.

- **Fiber is your friend!** Smoothies have fiber, juices don't. So a smoothie is a better option than juice if you're trying to lose weight. The fiber in your smoothie regulates the intake of natural sugars and keeps you fuller longer, making it easier to avoid hunger or cravings.

If your family needs a little encouragement to get on the green smoothies bandwagon, check out www.dummies.com/extras/greensmoothies for ideas to make green smoothies work for the whole family.

In this part . . .

- ✔ Discover green smoothie recipes designed to help improve your overall health and appearance.

- ✔ Target your body's needs when facing chronic or serious medical conditions and find the right green smoothies to help you recover quicker.

- ✔ Power up your workout with green smoothie recipes designed to provide the necessary boost both before and after exercise.

- ✔ Prepare your body for pregnancy with green smoothie recipes for fertility, and then support you and your baby's health with green smoothie recipes for pregnancy and breast feeding.

- ✔ Find out if you're a good candidate for doing a detox with green smoothies, and get the lowdown on your detox options, complete with instructions and recipes.

Chapter 12

Green Smoothies for a Healthier You

In This Chapter

▶ Understanding how diet impacts your health

▶ Finding relief from acid reflux symptoms

▶ Uncovering better skin with the help of a better diet

▶ Blending fiber-rich smoothies to help with digestive health

▶ Creating better diet habits for long-term weight loss success

*E*ven minor issues like skin eruptions, acid reflux, constipation, or weight gain can take their toll on your energy levels, sleep function, self-esteem, and general well-being. Long-term, some of these conditions can lead to more serious health problems like diabetes and cardiovascular disease. Finding relief of your symptoms through natural foods can help to reverse your condition, get you feeling better faster, and even boost your immune system for life.

This chapter addresses the most common health complaints that you may be suffering from and offers specialized green smoothie recipes to help bring your body back to balance, naturally. When you're facing a minor ailment, refer to this chapter to find out which green smoothie recipe is best for you. If you have a friend or loved one who is suffering from acid reflux, constipation, rashes, or skin problems, find the corresponding recipes for his condition in this chapter and offer him a helping hand by making a green smoothie for his health. You may be surprised at how quickly you can see and experience positive results!

The Apple Cider Vinegar and Bee Pollen Tonic smoothie recipe in this chapter calls for bee pollen, which you should leave out if you're allergic to pollen or to bees. Even if you don't have one of these allergies, before including that ingredient in a smoothie flip to Chapter 6 for info on how to determine whether you're sensitive to consuming bee pollen.

> **Recipes in This Chapter (cont.)**
>
> ▶ Slimming Apple Lemon Celery Blend
>
> ▶ Energy-Boosting Blackberry and Mint
>
> ▶ Strawberry Vanilla Healthy Indulgence
>
> ▶ Cucumber and Melon Natural Slender
>
> ▶ Dazzling Passion Fruit, Papaya, and Cinnamon
>
> ▶ Watermelon Kiwi Lime Creation
>
>

Cooling the Burn of Acid Reflux

If you start to feel queasy just from looking at a hot pepper, the smoothies in this section are definitely for you. *Acid reflux* and *heartburn* are common terms used to describe what is actually known as *esophagusburn.* Technically speaking, when you have heartburn, it's your *esophagus,* the channel that carries food to your stomach, that's on fire and not your heart. The problem actually lies in your gut.

Acid reflux occurs when the acids in the stomach start reversing, or *refluxing,* from the stomach back up the throat. Reflux causes a very uncomfortable burning sensation and a lot of discomfort. Having more than two episodes of heartburn per week can lead to more chronic and serious conditions such as GERD (gastroesophageal reflux disease) and gastric ulcers.

The fact that the antacid industry is booming shows you what a growing problem acid reflux has become. Prescription medications for reflux are in the three highest selling classes of drugs. Taking a pill every day for the rest of your life doesn't solve the problem; it only takes away the symptom. With the underlying issue still there, you leave yourself at a higher risk for developing other diseases down the line, including digestive disorders such as irritable bowel syndrome (IBS) and even certain types of cancer.

What's the main cause of acid reflux? Diet! Here are some ways to combat or prevent reflux:

✔ Keep your plate clear of fried food, refined food, processed food, and fatty meats, and don't overeat.

✔ Reduce or eliminate alcohol, tobacco, coffee, and sugary drinks.

✔ Drink plenty of water between meals.

When you change your diet, your symptoms should automatically start to decrease. Adding one healing green smoothie to your daily routine helps your stomach begin to repair and rebalance to its normal healthy acid levels.

 Foods known to help relieve acid reflux include cantaloupe, honeydew, banana, mango, fennel, parsley, carob, and ginger, as well as small amounts of fresh lemon juice, raw apple cider vinegar, and mint.

 Pregnant women commonly experience heartburn during pregnancy; however, the recipes in this section aren't recommended for pregnant or breast-feeding mothers. You can find green smoothie recipes for pregnancy in Chapter 15.

Raw cacao powder versus carob powder

Both cacao and carob are chocolate-like health foods, so people sometimes confuse them. But each has distinct characteristics and uses. Here's a breakdown:

Cacao powder:

✔ Made from the seeds of cacao fruit grown on the cacao tree; thrives in climates with high humidity and rainfall, like Central and South America

✔ Has a more bitter taste, like dark chocolate

✔ Contains caffeine and theobromine, both of which provide a stimulating effect

✔ Boasts higher amounts of iron, copper, magnesium, and manganese than carob does

✔ High in immune-boosting antioxidants

✔ Considered a superfood (flip to Chapter 6)

Carob powder:

✔ Comes from the pod of a carob tree; grown in dry climates and native to the eastern Mediterranean region

✔ Has a mild, naturally sweet taste somewhat similar to milk chocolate but without the sugar or milk

✔ Free of both caffeine and theobromine, offering a more calming effect than cacao powder does

✔ High in nutrients and a good vegan source of protein

✔ Suitable alternative for anyone who is intolerant to caffeine or has an allergy to chocolate

As you can see, it's not really a matter of choosing the best one because both cacao and carob powder offer health benefits. Use cacao powder when you're looking to jump-start your energy and elevate your mood. Opt for carob powder when you want a more calming effect on digestion, mood, or energy levels.

Soothing Pear, Mint, and Ginger

Prep time: 3 min • **Blending time:** 2 min • **Yield:** 3 servings

Ingredients	Directions
3 ripe pears	*1* Cut the pears and remove the core, keeping the skin intact. Cut the flesh into quarters.
½-inch piece fresh ginger (peeled)	
1 tablespoon fresh lime juice	*2* Combine the pears, ginger, lime juice, flax-seed, and water in the blender and secure the lid.
1 tablespoon ground flaxseed	
2½ cups water	*3* Starting at low speed and gradually increasing toward high, blend the ingredients for 15 to 30 seconds or until the mixture contains no visible pieces of fruit.
4 mint leaves	
2 cups celery leaves, loosely packed	
1 cup baby spinach, loosely packed	*4* Add the mint, celery leaves, and spinach and blend again at medium speed for 30 seconds, gradually increasing the speed to high. Blend on high speed for another 15 seconds or until the entire mixture is smooth.
	5 Pour the smoothie into two glasses and enjoy!

Per serving: Calories 203 (From Fat 18); Fat 2g (Saturated 0g); Cholesterol 0mg; Sodium 109mg; Carbohydrate 48g (Dietary Fiber 11g); Protein 4g.

Tip: If you don't like the taste of mint, you can leave out the mint leaves. If you don't have fresh ginger available, substitute ¼ teaspoon of ground ginger.

Parsley, Mango, and Apple Vinegar Tonic

Prep time: 3–4 min • **Blending time:** 2 min • **Yield:** 2 servings

Ingredients	Directions
1 ripe mango	*1* Peel the mango and cut the flesh away from the stone.
1 ripe banana, peeled	
1½ cups water	*2* Combine all ingredients except the parsley in the blender and secure the lid.
2 tablespoons raw apple cider vinegar	
2 cups parsley, loosely packed	*3* Starting at low speed and gradually increasing toward high, blend the ingredients for 1 minute or until smooth.
	4 Add the parsley and blend again at medium speed for 30 to 45 seconds, gradually increasing the speed to high. Blend on high speed for another 15 seconds or until the entire mixture is smooth.
	5 Pour the smoothie into two glasses and enjoy!

Per serving: Calories 136 (From Fat 9); Fat 1g (Saturated 0g); Cholesterol 0mg; Sodium 41mg; Carbohydrate 33g (Dietary Fiber 5g); Protein 3g.

Tip: Reduce the amount of raw apple cider vinegar to ½ tablespoon per smoothie (1 tablespoon total) if you have acid reflux more than twice a week. As you drink more smoothies over time, you rebuild your normal stomach acids and strengthen digestion, so you can slowly increase to 2 tablespoons.

Tip: If you don't have raw apple cider vinegar, use 2 tablespoons of fresh lime juice instead.

Warning: Don't use raw apple cider vinegar if you have stomach ulcers.

Ginger, Grape, and Lemon Elixir

Prep time: 3–4 min • **Blending time:** 2 min • **Yield:** 2 servings

Ingredients	Directions
1½ cups red or green grapes	**1** Combine all the ingredients except the spinach in the blender and secure the lid.
1 ripe banana, peeled	
½-inch piece fresh ginger (peeled)	**2** Starting at low speed and gradually increasing toward high, blend the ingredients for 30 to 45 seconds or until the mixture contains no visible pieces of fruit.
2 tablespoons fresh lemon juice	
1½ cups water	**3** Add the spinach and blend again at medium speed for 30 seconds, gradually increasing the speed to high. Blend on high speed for another 15 to 30 seconds or until the entire mixture is smooth.
2 cups baby spinach, loosely packed	
	4 Pour the smoothie into two glasses and enjoy!

Per serving: Calories 165 (From Fat 9); Fat 1g (Saturated 0g); Cholesterol 0mg; Sodium 36mg; Carbohydrate 41g (Dietary Fiber 3g); Protein 3g.

Tip: If you don't have fresh ginger, use ¼ teaspoon of ground ginger instead.

Tip: Leave out the lemon juice if you suffer from really bad heartburn. Over time, as your body becomes stronger and more in balance, you can add lemon juice slowly, starting with 1 tablespoon and gradually increasing to 2 tablespoons total (that's 1 tablespoon per smoothie). Believe it or not, small amounts of lemon juice are actually good for digestion and can help relieve symptoms of milder heartburn.

Vary It! Instead of grapes, use 2 kiwis (peeled) or 1 pear (cored and quartered with the skin intact).

Cool ABC: Aloe Vera, Banana, and Carob

Prep time: 25 min • **Blending time:** 2 min • **Yield:** 2 servings

Ingredients	Directions
2 tablespoons chia seeds	*1* Place the chia seeds in a bowl with ¼ cup of room temperature water. Place in the fridge to soak for at least 20 minutes or overnight.
2 Medjool dates, pitted	
2 ripe bananas, peeled	
2 tablespoons raw honey	*2* Combine all the ingredients except the spinach in the blender and secure the lid.
1 teaspoon carob powder	
2 tablespoons aloe vera juice	*3* Starting at low speed and gradually increasing toward high, blend the ingredients for 30 to 45 seconds or until the mixture contains no visible pieces of fruit.
1½ cups water	
2 cups baby spinach, loosely packed	
	4 Add the spinach and blend again at medium speed for 30 seconds, gradually increasing the speed to high. Blend on high speed for another 15 to 30 seconds or until the entire mixture is smooth.
	5 Pour the smoothie into two glasses. Enjoy!

Per serving: Calories 325 (From Fat 45); Fat 5g (Saturated 0.5g); Cholesterol 0mg; Sodium 32mg; Carbohydrate 73g (Dietary Fiber 11g); Protein 5g.

Tip: Carob sometimes functions as a chocolate replacement, but don't replace carob powder with raw cacao powder for this recipe. Carob powder is known to calm the effects of acid reflux, whereas cacao powder can actually make it worse.

Vary It! Add 1 apple (cored and quartered), 1 pear (cored and quartered), or 1 cup of green or red grapes for a fruitier flavor.

Apple Fennel Relief

Prep time: 3–4 min • **Blending time:** 2 min • **Yield:** 2 servings

Ingredients	*Directions*
2 red apples	***1*** Cut the apples and remove the core, keeping the skin intact. Cut the flesh into quarters.
1 ripe banana, peeled	
½ teaspoon ground fennel seed	***2*** Combine all the ingredients except the kale in the blender and secure the lid.
1 tablespoon raw honey	
1 drop pure peppermint oil	***3*** Starting at low speed and gradually increasing toward high, blend the ingredients for 30 to 45 seconds or until the mixture contains no visible pieces of fruit.
1½ cups water	
2 large kale leaves	
	4 Remove and discard the stems of the kale. Add the kale and blend again at medium speed for 30 seconds, gradually increasing the speed to high. Blend on high speed for another 15 to 30 seconds or until the entire mixture is smooth.
	5 Pour the smoothie into two glasses and enjoy!

Per serving: Calories 206 (From Fat 9); Fat 1g (Saturated 0g); Cholesterol 0mg; Sodium 21mg; Carbohydrate 50g (Dietary Fiber 7g); Protein 3g.

Tip: If you have access to fresh fennel, use ¼ cup chopped fresh fennel instead of the ground fennel. If you don't like the taste of peppermint, you can omit the peppermint oil.

Vary It! Use 1½ cups of red or green grapes instead of apple.

Basil, Peach, and Honeydew

Prep time: 3–4 min • **Blending time:** 2 min • **Yield:** 2 servings

Ingredients	Directions
1 ripe peach	**1** Cut the peach and remove the core, keeping the skin intact. Cut the flesh into quarters.
2 cups chopped honeydew	
1 tablespoon raw honey	**2** Combine the peach, honeydew, honey, and water in the blender and secure the lid.
1½ cups water	
4 basil leaves	**3** Starting at low speed and gradually increasing toward high, blend the ingredients for 30 to 45 seconds or until the mixture contains no visible pieces of fruit (although you will see some of the peach skin).
1 cup baby spinach, loosely packed	
	4 Add the basil and spinach and blend again at medium speed for 30 seconds, gradually increasing the speed to high. Blend on high speed for another 15 to 30 seconds or until the entire mixture is smooth.
	5 Pour the smoothie into two glasses and enjoy!

Per serving: Calories 128 (From Fat 4); Fat 0.5g (Saturated 0g); Cholesterol 0mg; Sodium 48mg; Carbohydrate 32g (Dietary Fiber 3g); Protein 2g.

Vary It! Use 4 fresh mint leaves instead of fresh basil. You can even try adding 4 leaves of both!

Eating Your Way to Fabulous Skin

When it comes to having beautiful skin, the age-old saying "you are what you eat" couldn't ring more true. Your skin is actually the largest organ in your body, and it's responsible not only for protecting your body from outside damage but also for expelling internal toxins and acid waste directly through its pores. In fact, your skin eliminates a quarter of your body's total waste every day.

While you're getting an adequate amount of sleep at night, your skin is working hard to get rid of metabolic impurities, flush out acids, and help cleanse your body from the inside out. Through the process of renewal and repair, your skin constantly sheds older cells and replaces them with new ones. You need a steady supply of vitamins, minerals, antioxidants, and alkaline-forming foods to support the new cell growth.

The foods you eat define how soft, smooth, and clear your skin will be. The following dietary factors contribute to common skin conditions such as acne, psoriasis, eczema, and rosacea:

- Too many refined carbohydrates such as white bread, pasta, and refined sugary treats

- Dairy, which generates internal mucous that can clog pores

- Fried foods, which are full of damaged molecules or *free radicals* that put the skin into overdrive

- Alcohol, which promotes inflammation that can trigger more breakouts and flare-ups

- Dehydration (not drinking enough water), which can leave the skin dry and unable to do its job

Tobacco use and overexposure to the sun add further damage to the skin, causing small wrinkles and age spots to appear over time. The term *anti-aging* is a bit misleading because you can't stop the hands of time, but through eating a better diet, you can slow down the damage to your skin's cells. Eating foods high in antioxidants — such as lemons, oranges, berries, mangoes, pineapples, and grapes — is an excellent path to clearer skin. Adding more dark leafy greens (especially watercress) to your diet gives you chlorophyll, another important nutrient for healthy skin. Other healing foods for skin include aloe vera, avocado, cucumber, and good sources of omega-3 fatty acids, such as flaxseeds and chia seeds.

Ageless Papaya and Blueberry

Prep time: 25 min • **Blending time:** 2 min • **Yield:** 2 servings

Ingredients	Directions
2 tablespoons chia seeds	*1* Place the chia seeds in a bowl with ¼ cup of room temperature water. Place in the fridge to soak for at least 20 minutes or overnight.
3 cups chopped papaya, seeded and peeled	
1 cup blueberries	
3 tablespoons fresh lime juice	*2* Combine all the ingredients except the spinach in the blender and secure the lid.
1½ cups water	
2 cups baby spinach, loosely packed	*3* Starting at low speed and gradually increasing toward high, blend the ingredients for 45 seconds or until the mixture contains no visible pieces of fruit.
	4 Add the spinach and blend again at medium speed for 30 seconds, gradually increasing the speed to high. Blend on high speed for another 15 to 30 seconds or until the entire mixture is smooth.
	5 Pour the smoothie into two glasses and enjoy!

Per serving: Calories 217 (From Fat 45); Fat 5g (Saturated 0.5g); Cholesterol 0mg; Sodium 47mg; Carbohydrate 42g (Dietary Fiber 11g); Protein 5g.

Tip: Add 2 tablespoons of soaked goji berries or 1 tablespoon of acai powder for more antioxidants.

Vary It! Add a dash of ground turmeric or ground cinnamon for a different twist. For a minty fresh flavor, add 3 or 4 mint leaves in Step 4.

Smooth Mango, Kiwi, and Watercress

Prep time: 3–4 min • **Blending time:** 2 min • **Yield:** 2 servings

Ingredients	Directions
1 ripe mango	**1** Peel the mango and cut the flesh away from the stone.
2 kiwis, peeled	
1 ripe banana, peeled	**2** Combine all the ingredients except the watercress in the blender and secure the lid.
2 tablespoons ground flaxseed	
1½ cups water	**3** Starting at low speed and gradually increasing toward high, blend the ingredients for 45 seconds or until the mixture contains no visible pieces of fruit.
2 cups watercress, loosely packed	
	4 Add the watercress and blend again at medium speed for 30 seconds, gradually increasing the speed to high. Blend on high speed for another 15 to 30 seconds or until the entire mixture is smooth.
	5 Pour the smoothie into two glasses and enjoy!

Per serving: Calories 195 (From Fat 27); Fat 3g (Saturated 0g); Cholesterol 0mg; Sodium 23mg; Carbohydrate 43g (Dietary Fiber 8g); Protein 5g.

Tip: Look for watercress greens either in loose form with other fresh greens or in a plastic container near the fresh herbs section in your grocery store.

Tip: If you don't have access to fresh mango, use 2 cups of pineapple chunks or 2 peaches (cored and quartered) instead.

Aloe Ginger Peachy Dandy

Prep time: 3–4 min • **Blending time:** 2 min • **Yield:** 2 servings

Ingredients	Directions
2 ripe peaches	*1* Cut the peaches and remove the stones, keeping the skin intact. Cut the flesh into quarters.
2 cups pineapple chunks	
2 tablespoons ground hemp seed	*2* Combine the peaches, pineapple, hemp seed, aloe vera, ginger, and water in the blender and secure the lid.
2 tablespoons aloe vera juice	
½-inch piece fresh ginger (peeled)	*3* Starting at low speed and gradually easing toward high, blend the ingredients for 1 minute or until smooth.
1½ cups water	
1 cup dandelion leaves, loosely packed	*4* Add the dandelion and celery leaves and blend again at medium speed for 45 seconds, gradually increasing the speed to high. Blend on high speed for another 15 to 30 seconds or until the entire mixture is smooth.
1 cup celery leaves, loosely packed	
	5 Pour the smoothie into two glasses and enjoy!

Per serving: Calories 336 (From Fat 72); Fat 8g (Saturated 1g); Cholesterol 0mg; Sodium 92mg; Carbohydrate 61g (Dietary Fiber 8g); Protein 8g.

Tip: If you don't have fresh ginger, use ¼ teaspoon of ground ginger instead. If you don't have fresh dandelion leaves at your local farmers' market, opt for mustard greens, beet greens, or parsnip greens instead.

Vary It! Add a peeled banana for a smoother, creamier texture.

Silky Pear and Avocado

Prep time: 25 min • **Blending time:** 2 min • **Yield:** 2 servings

Ingredients	Directions
2 tablespoons chia seeds 1 ripe pear 1 red delicious or gala apple	**1** Place the chia seeds in a bowl with ¼ cup of room temperature water. Place in the fridge to soak for at least 20 minutes or overnight.
½ avocado, peeled and pitted 1 tablespoon fresh lemon juice	**2** Cut the pear and apple and remove the cores, keeping the skin intact. Cut the flesh into quarters.
2 Medjool dates, pitted 1½ cups water 2 large romaine lettuce leaves	**3** Add the all the ingredients except the lettuce and spinach to the blender and secure the lid.
1 cup baby spinach, loosely packed	**4** Starting at low speed and gradually increasing toward high, blend the ingredients for 1 minute or until the mixture contains no visible pieces of fruit.
	5 Add the lettuce and spinach and blend again at medium speed for 30 to 45 seconds, gradually increasing the speed to high. Blend on high speed for another 15 seconds or until the entire mixture is smooth.
	6 Pour the smoothie into two glasses and enjoy!

Per serving: Calories 299 (From Fat 90); Fat 10g (Saturated 1g); Cholesterol 0mg; Sodium 25mg; Carbohydrate 54g (Dietary Fiber 15g); Protein 5g.

Apple Cider Vinegar and Bee Pollen Tonic

Prep time: 3–4 min • **Blending time:** 2 min • **Yield:** 2 servings

Ingredients	Directions
1 green apple	*1* Cut the apple and remove the core, keeping the skin intact. Cut the flesh into quarters.
2 cups red or green grapes	
1 ripe banana, peeled	
3 tablespoons raw apple cider vinegar	*2* Add the apple, grapes, banana, apple cider vinegar, acai powder, bee pollen, and water to the blender and secure the lid.
1 tablespoon acai powder	
1 tablespoon bee pollen (omit if allergic)	*3* Starting at low speed and gradually increasing toward high, blend the ingredients for 1 minute or until the mixture contains no visible pieces of fruit.
1½ cups water	
1 cup parsley, loosely packed	
1 cup watercress, loosely packed	*4* Add the parsley and watercress and blend again at medium speed for 30 to 45 seconds, gradually increasing the speed to high. Blend on high speed for another 15 seconds or until the entire mixture is smooth.
	5 Pour the smoothie into two glasses and enjoy!

Per serving: Calories 248 (From Fat 18); Fat 2g (Saturated 0.5g); Cholesterol 0mg; Sodium 34mg; Carbohydrate 59g (Dietary Fiber 7g); Protein 5g.

Tip: Check the label of your apple cider vinegar to make sure it's raw. It should read "unpasteurized" or "with the mother." Refer to the sidebar "Benefits of raw apple cider vinegar" earlier in this chapter for more on the health benefits of raw apple cider vinegar.

Orange and Melon Perfection

Prep time: 3–4 min • **Blending time:** 2 min • **Yield:** 2 servings

Ingredients	*Directions*
3 cups chopped cantaloupe 1 orange, peeled and seeded 2 tablespoons aloe vera juice 2 tablespoons ground flaxseed 1½ cups water 3 large kale leaves	*1* Combine all the ingredients except the kale in the blender and secure the lid. Starting at a low speed and gradually increasing toward high, blend the ingredients for 30 to 45 seconds or until the mixture contains no visible pieces of fruit. *2* Remove and discard the stems of the kale. Add the kale and blend again at medium speed for 30 seconds, gradually increasing the speed to high. Blend on high speed for another 15 to 30 seconds or until the entire mixture is smooth. *3* Pour the smoothie into two glasses and enjoy!

Per serving: Calories 167 (From Fat 27); Fat 3g (Saturated 0g); Cholesterol 0mg; Sodium 57mg; Carbohydrate 34g (Dietary Fiber 6g); Protein 6g.

Vary It! Add ½-inch piece of fresh ginger for a more robust flavor, 3 or 4 fresh mint leaves for a fresh twist, or even 2 tablespoons of raw honey for a sweeter taste.

Minimizing skin damage: Oxidation

Have you ever noticed how an apple starts turning brown just minutes after you cut it? When the cells inside the apple are exposed to oxygen, the apple starts to break down. That damage is a process called *oxidative stress*. On a much slower scale, the same thing is happening to you, both internally and externally. When you're young, your skin is clear, soft, and supple. As the years go by, you notice new wrinkles, sagging skin, or age spots until all of a sudden, your skin is noticeably aged. Chemical body products, prescription drugs, recreational drugs, alcohol, tobacco, smog, excess sunlight, and stress all add fuel to the oxidative fire. Throw in a diet full of processed or fried foods, and you've just fast-tracked your oxidation rate.

To avoid oxidative stress, you need a diet high in antioxidants to neutralize any free radical damage in your body and stop oxidation from spreading. Choosing foods high in antioxidants helps to minimize the effects of aging and decrease your risk of major diseases such as heart disease, cancer, autoimmune disease, fibromyalgia, arthritis, and macular degeneration. It's that simple! Antioxidants occur in all fresh fruits and vegetables (especially berries, pineapples, avocados, lemons, oranges, apples, and all dark leafy bitter greens) as well as goji berries and acai powder.

Finding Relief from Constipation

Unfortunately, nature doesn't always call like you hope it will. If you suffer from constipation, you know that what goes in doesn't always come out, at least not right away. *Constipation* happens when solid waste (stool) spends too much time in your colon. The colon absorbs too much water from the stool, making the stool hard, dry, and difficult to pass.

Constipation can make you feel tired, bloated, gassy, weak, toxic, irritable, and uncomfortable. It can give you bad breath and some-times cause significant abdominal pain. Over time, chronic consti-pation can lead to chronic colon inflammation, which contributes to a higher risk of certain types of colon cancer. Basically, the sooner things move, the better.

What actually constitutes true constipation? Like many things, it depends on whom you ask. Some experts claim that having a bowel movement three times per week is enough, while others insist that you should be going at least once a day (and twice is better). You know you're constipated if

- ✔ Your stool is hard or difficult to pass
- ✔ You have to sit on the toilet more than 3 minutes
- ✔ Your stool consists of very small pellets

I like to observe animals in nature for the simplest and most logi-cal understanding. And guess what? They're going every day, at least once and sometimes two or three times a day. The difference is that animals in nature aren't eating refined, fiber-lacking foods such as donuts, fried everything, and ice cream. (Well, unless it's a bear digging in a dumpster somewhere, and I can guarantee that he'll have a definite back-up in the pipes after that!) They're eating lots of plant-based foods, meaning plenty of fruits, vegetables, and especially greens. All those foods are full of fiber, and fiber is the broom that gets things moving. Fresh fruits and vegetables are also full of valuable enzymes that help break food down for digestion.

Other causes of constipation include

- ✔ Lack of physical activity
- ✔ Stress
- ✔ Lack of good bacteria in the gut
- ✔ Not drinking enough water

✔ Ignoring the urge to go

✔ Side effects from certain medications

Having a fiber-rich green smoothie is the best way to keep nature calling regularly. Specific foods that help relieve constipation include papayas, pineapples, persimmons, dates, bananas, pears, prunes, figs, peaches, nectarines, apricots, flaxseeds, and chia seeds. In addition to bumping up your fiber intake, try the following suggestions to improve your overall colon health:

✔ **Add more variety to your diet.** Try not to eat the same foods every day.

✔ **Eat a rainbow of colors.** A range of colors means you're bringing in a range of different minerals and enzymes to give your gut a good workout.

✔ **Drink more water.** A lot of constipation occurs from simple dehydration!

✔ **Increase exercise.** Go for a brisk walk or take a stretching class.

✔ **Listen to your gut.** Don't ignore the urge to go!

Adding probiotics for good gut bacteria

A healthy digestive system has a balance of good bacteria versus bad bacteria. Good bacteria bring plenty of oxygen to the colon, helping create a healthy, disease-free environment in the gut. Bad bacteria take away oxygen, which creates a toxic, decaying, foul-smelling mess — the perfect breeding ground for disease. Antibiotics tend to kill all bacteria, so they open the door for the bad guys to take over.

If you suffer from constipation and have a history of taking antibiotics, taking one probiotic supplement daily is an easy, natural way to get good bacteria back in your gut for better colon health. *Probiotic* means "healthful to life," and that's exactly what good bacteria are to your body! To make things really easy, add a probiotic capsule to your green smoothie. Just throw it in there and blend! If you prefer, you can simply take the capsule while drinking your smoothie.

Note: You may have heard of acidophilis; that's one type of probiotic found in yogurt. The problem with yogurt is that it's totally lacking in dietary fiber and often also contains added refined sugar. Your best bet is to take a probiotic in capsule form. Look for it in the refrigerated section of your local health food store.

Papaya and Pineapple Remedy

Prep time: 4–5 min • **Blending time:** 2 min • **Yield:** 2 servings

Ingredients	*Directions*
1½ cups pineapple chunks 1½ cups chopped papaya, seeded and peeled 1 tablespoon fresh lime juice 2 tablespoons ground flaxseed 1 tablespoon coconut oil 1½ cups water 1 cup parsley, loosely packed 1 cup bok choy leaves, loosely packed	*1* Combine the pineapple, papaya, lime juice, flaxseed, coconut oil, and water in the blender and secure the lid. *2* Starting at low speed and gradually increasing toward high, blend the ingredients for 1 minute or until the mixture contains no visible pieces of fruit. *3* Add the parsley and bok choy and blend again at medium speed for 30 seconds, gradually increasing the speed to high. Blend on high speed for another 15 to 30 seconds or until the entire mixture is smooth. *4* Pour the smoothie into 2 glasses and enjoy!

Per serving: Calories 256 (From Fat 90); Fat 10g (Saturated 6g); Cholesterol 0mg; Sodium 69mg; Carbohydrate 42g (Dietary Fiber 7g); Protein 3g.

Tip: Add half a ripe banana for a smoother and creamier texture.

Vary It! Try fresh mango instead of papaya.

Persimmon Power

Prep time: 3–4 min • **Blending time:** 2 min • **Yield:** 2 servings

Ingredients	Directions
2 ripe persimmons	*1* Cut the persimmons and remove the stems and any large seeds, keeping the skin intact. Cut the flesh into quarters.
1 ripe banana, peeled	
1 orange, peeled and seeded	
½-inch piece fresh ginger (peeled)	*2* Combine all the ingredients except the kale in the blender and secure the lid.
1½ cups water	*3* Starting at low speed and gradually increasing toward high, blend the ingredients for 30 to 45 seconds or until the mixture contains no visible pieces of fruit.
4 large kale leaves	
	4 Remove and discard the stems of the kale. Add the kale and blend again at medium speed for 30 seconds, gradually increasing the speed to high. Blend on high speed for another 15 to 30 seconds or until the entire mixture is smooth.
	5 Pour the smoothie into two glasses and enjoy!

Per serving: Calories 156 (From Fat 9); Fat 1g (Saturated 0g); Cholesterol 0mg; Sodium 24mg; Carbohydrate 37g (Dietary Fiber 4g); Protein 4g.

Tip: Not all persimmons have large seeds, but some varieties do. If you don't see any large black seeds when you cut open the fruit, you don't need to remove anything except the stem.

Tip: Sprinkle the smoothie with a dash of ground cinnamon before serving for an added sweet flavor.

Vary It! Replace the ginger with ½ teaspoon of ground turmeric.

Date with Nectarine and Strawberry

Prep time: 25 min • **Blending time:** 2 min • **Yield:** 2 servings

Ingredients	Directions
2 tablespoons chia seeds 4 ripe nectarines 1½ cups halved strawberries, stems and leaves removed 1 Medjool date, pitted 1 tablespoon coconut oil 1 tablespoon raw cacao powder 1½ cups water 2 large collard green leaves	**1** Place the chia seeds in a bowl with ¼ cup of room temperature water. Place in the fridge to soak for at least 20 minutes or overnight. **2** Cut the nectarines and remove the stones, keeping the skin intact. Cut the flesh into quarters. **3** Add all the ingredients except the collard greens to the blender and secure the lid. **4** Starting at low speed and gradually increasing toward high, blend the ingredients for 1 minute or until the mixture contains no visible pieces of fruit. **5** Add the collard greens and blend again at medium speed for 45 seconds, gradually increasing the speed to high. Blend on high speed for another 15 to 30 seconds or until the entire mixture is smooth. **6** Pour the smoothie into two glasses and enjoy!

Per serving: Calories 391 (From Fat 117); Fat 13g (Saturated 7g); Cholesterol 0mg; Sodium 11mg; Carbohydrate 64g (Dietary Fiber 16g); Protein 9g.

Tip: If you can't find fresh nectarines, use fresh peaches instead. You can also use 4 tablespoons of ground flaxseed if you don't have chia seeds.

Vary It! Replace the water and coconut oil with 1½ cups of coconut water.

Fast-Acting Pear and Prunes

Prep time: 3–4 min • **Blending time:** 2 min • **Yield:** 2 servings

Ingredients	Directions
2 ripe pears 6 pitted prunes 1 ripe banana, peeled 2 tablespoons ground flaxseed Dash of vanilla extract Dash of ground cinnamon 1½ cups water 3 Swiss chard leaves	*1* Cut the pears and remove the cores, keeping the skin intact. Cut the flesh into quarters. *2* Combine all the ingredients except the Swiss chard in the blender and secure the lid. *3* Starting at low speed and gradually increasing toward high, blend the ingredients for 30 to 45 seconds or until the mixture contains no visible pieces of fruit. *4* Remove and discard the stems of the Swiss chard. Add the Swiss chard and blend again at medium speed for 30 seconds, gradually increasing the speed to high. Blend on high speed for another 15 to 30 seconds or until the entire mixture is smooth. *5* Pour the smoothie into two glasses and enjoy!

Per serving: Calories 256 (From Fat 27); Fat 3g (Saturated 0g); Cholesterol 0mg; Sodium 47mg; Carbohydrate 60g (Dietary Fiber 11g); Protein 4g.

Tip: If plums are in season, add 2 ripe plums (stones removed) instead of prunes.

Vary It! Use 2 peeled kiwis instead of 2 pears for a different taste. Add a dash of ground cardamom instead of cinnamon.

Cinnamon Fig-Lax

Prep time: 25 min • **Blending time:** 2 min • **Yield:** 2 servings

Ingredients	Directions
2 teaspoons chia seeds	*1* Place the chia seeds in a bowl with ¼ cup of room temperature water. Place in the fridge to soak for at least 20 minutes or overnight.
6 fresh figs, stems removed and quartered	
2 ripe bananas, peeled	*2* Combine all the ingredients except the spinach in the blender and secure the lid.
½ teaspoon ground cinnamon	
1½ cups water	*3* Starting at low speed and gradually increasing toward high, blend the ingredients for 30 to 45 seconds or until the mixture contains no visible pieces of fruit.
2 cups baby spinach, loosely packed	
	4 Add the spinach and blend again at medium speed for 30 seconds, gradually increasing the speed to high. Blend on high speed for another 15 to 30 seconds or until the entire mixture is smooth.
	5 Pour the smoothie into two glasses and enjoy!

Per serving: Calories 297 (From Fat 45); Fat 5g (Saturated 1g); Cholesterol 0mg; Sodium 32mg; Carbohydrate 64g (Dietary Fiber 14g); Protein 6g.

Tip: Substitute 4 dried figs soaked in water for 20 minutes if you can't get fresh figs. If you soak dried figs before blending, they blend better and add a creamier texture to the smoothie.

Vary It! Add a dash of ground cardamom instead of cinnamon.

Cherry, Apricot, and Aloe Accelerator

Prep time: 3–4 min • **Blending time:** 2 min • **Yield:** 2 servings

Ingredients	Directions
4 ripe apricots	*1* Cut the apricots and remove the stones, keeping the skin intact. Cut the flesh into quarters.
1½ cups cherries, pitted	
1 Medjool date, pitted	
2 tablespoons aloe vera juice	*2* Combine all the ingredients except the romaine in the blender and secure the lid.
2 tablespoons ground flaxseed	
1½ cups water	*3* Starting at low speed and gradually increasing toward high, blend the ingredients for 30 to 45 seconds or until the mixture contains no visible pieces of fruit.
4 romaine lettuce leaves	
	4 Add the lettuce and blend again at medium speed for 30 seconds, gradually increasing the speed to high. Blend on high speed for another 15 to 30 seconds or until the entire mixture is smooth.
	5 Pour the smoothie into two glasses and enjoy!

Per serving: Calories 165 (From Fat 27); Fat 3g (Saturated 0g); Cholesterol 0mg; Sodium 8mg; Carbohydrate 33g (Dietary Fiber 5g); Protein 5g.

Tip: You can substitute 8 dried organic apricots (soaked in water for 20 minutes) for the fresh apricots. If you can't find fresh cherries, look for unsweetened cherry juice from your local health food store. Add 1 cup of cherry juice instead of the fresh cherries.

Vary It! Use 2 fresh peaches (stones removed) instead of cherries, or add both!

Achieving Goals with Weight Loss

Overall, the obesity statistics aren't telling a good tale. Until now, the bulge has been winning the battle, and the next generation is shaping up to be Generation XXL. Obesity can be a serious health issue, bringing increased risk of every type of disease, including diabetes, heart disease, high blood pressure, high cholesterol, and even certain types of cancer.

Of course, not every overweight person is obese. But even if you only have a few excess pounds to shed, losing weight can still be tough. No matter how much you want to lose, finding real success with weight loss is never easy.

The most common obstacles you may face are

✔ Not having enough time to prepare healthy food

✔ Feeling overwhelmed with having to learn new recipes

✔ Worrying about feeling hungry or unsatisfied

✔ Lacking the motivation to try *another* new diet

Adding a green smoothie can definitely help! Let your green smoothie complement your current diet and shine new light on a healthy way of living. With a blender, fresh ingredients, and less than five minutes, you solve all those problems and you have an easy, fiber-rich replacement meal or afternoon snack to keep away the hunger. Where there's a green smoothie, there's hope!

To make the best green smoothies for weight loss, consider the following points:

✔ **Increase the amount of water.** More water gives you more smoothie! Get the feeling of eating more and dilute the natural sugars in your smoothie by simply adding more water. You can use 2 to 3 cups of water instead of the normal 1½ cups during a weight loss regimen.

✔ **Choose fruits with high water content.** Try grapes, apples, peaches, plums, papaya, watermelon, and pears. Add a bit of citrus, such as fresh lemon or lime juice, or raw apple cider vinegar to help speed digestion.

✔ **Use bananas in moderation.** Banana is an excellent high-fiber fruit, but it also packs a few calories. To lose weight, use bananas sparingly in smoothies (no more than half a banana at a time) and spread your caloric load throughout the day.

✔ **Reduce the amount of flaxseed.** Adding 1 tablespoon of flaxseeds instead of 2 tablespoons minimizes added calories. If you're extra strict with calories, replace flaxseed or chia seeds with 1 or 2 tablespoons of psyllium husk powder.

✔ **Cut back on fatty ingredients.** Good fats are good but you can definitely have too many when trying to lose weight. You don't want too many fat calories in a smoothie; you won't even notice the difference without them. For example, coconut oil has a whopping 117 calories in just 1 tablespoon, so you should avoid using it during weight loss. Similarly, opt for smoothies without avocado and nuts.

Combining a balanced, healthy diet with regular exercise is the key to long-term weight loss success. Drink your green smoothie, but also get active for at least 20 to 30 minutes every day. The more lean muscle you have, the better your body is at burning fuel.

Adding more fiber: Bulk up to slim down

Fiber is the part of plant-based foods that humans can't digest. Most plant foods are a mix of soluble and insoluble fiber. *Soluble fiber* helps the body absorb nutrients from food, and *insoluble fiber* helps move food through the gut. Animal-based foods such as meat, cheese, yogurt, milk, and eggs contain no fiber.

A high-fiber diet has been shown to help control blood sugar levels in Type 2 diabetics, manage constipation, and improve symptoms of irritable bowel syndrome (IBS). Fiber can also help keep your weight in check by making you feel fuller.

Here's how you can work more fiber into your diet:

✔ **Stop peeling.** Leave the skin on fruits and vegetables; the skin is full of fiber!

✔ **Opt for seeds in smoothies.** Use flaxseed, psyllium powder, or chia seeds in your green smoothie.

✔ **Eat beans.** Add lentils, chickpeas, or black beans to a soup, salad, or main dish.

✔ **Snack smart.** Choose veggie sticks or whole, unsalted nuts and seeds.

Slimming Apple Lemon Celery Blend

Prep time: 3–4 min • **Blending time:** 2 min • **Yield:** 2 servings

Ingredients	Directions
1 red delicious or gala apple 1 green apple	**1** Cut the apples and remove the cores, keeping the skin intact.
1 orange, peeled and seeded ¼ cup fresh lemon juice 2 tablespoons raw apple cider vinegar	**2** Combine the apples, orange, lemon juice, vinegar, flaxseed, and water in the blender and secure the lid.
1 tablespoon ground flaxseed 2 cups water 5 mint leaves	**3** Starting at low speed and gradually increasing toward high, blend the ingredients for 30 to 45 seconds or until the mixture contains no visible pieces of fruit.
1½ cups celery leaves, loosely packed ½ cup parsley, loosely packed	**4** Add the mint, celery, and parsley and blend again at medium speed for 30 seconds, gradually increasing the speed to high. Blend on high speed for another 30 seconds or until the entire mixture is smooth.
	5 Pour the smoothie into two glasses and enjoy!

Per serving: Calories 187 (From Fat 27); Fat 3g (Saturated 0g); Cholesterol 0mg; Sodium 79mg; Carbohydrate 42g (Dietary Fiber 10g); Protein 4g.

Vary It! Add ¼ teaspoon of ground cinnamon for a warm, spicy flavor. You can also replace the orange with 2 cups of peeled chopped cucumber.

Energy-Boosting Blackberry and Mint

Prep time: 3–4 min • **Blending time:** 2 min • **Yield:** 2 servings

Ingredients	Directions
2 ripe pears	*1* Cut the pears and remove the cores, keeping the skin intact.
1½ cups blackberries	
½ cup fresh lime juice	*2* Combine the pears, blackberries, lime juice, hemp seed, psyllium powder, and water to the blender and secure the lid.
1 tablespoon ground hemp seed	
1 tablespoon psyllium husk powder	*3* Starting at low speed and gradually increasing toward high, blend the ingredients for 30 to 45 seconds or until the mixture contains no visible pieces of fruit.
2 cups water	
3 large kale leaves	
½ cup mint leaves	*4* Remove and discard the stems of the kale. Add the kale and mint and blend again at medium speed for 30 seconds, gradually increasing the speed to high. Blend on high speed for another 15 to 30 seconds or until the entire mixture is smooth.
	5 Pour the smoothie into two glasses and enjoy!

Per serving: Calories 232 (From Fat 45); Fat 5g (Saturated 0.5g); Cholesterol 0mg; Sodium 26mg; Carbohydrate 48g (Dietary Fiber 16g); Protein 7g.

Tip: You can use 1 drop of pure peppermint oil instead of fresh mint leaves.

Vary It! Use blueberries or raspberries instead of blackberries. During summer, use 1 ripe mango (peeled and stone removed) instead of pears.

Smoothies trump juices for weight loss

A smoothie (with fiber) is a better option than juice (with no fiber) if you're trying to lose weight. The fiber in your smoothie is what regulates your intake of natural sugars and keeps you fuller longer, which helps you avoid hunger and cravings. Chapter 1 has more info on the difference between a smoothie and a juice.

Strawberry Vanilla Healthy Indulgence

Prep time: 25 min • **Blending time:** 2 min • **Yield:** 2 servings

Ingredients	Directions
2 tablespoons chia seeds 2 ripe peaches 1 ripe plum 1½ cups halved strawberries, stems and leaves removed ½-inch piece fresh ginger (peeled) ¼ teaspoon vanilla extract Dash cayenne pepper 2 cups water 4 large Swiss chard leaves	*1* Place the chia seeds in a bowl with ¼ cup of room temperature water. Place in the fridge to soak for at least 20 minutes or overnight. *2* Cut the peaches and plum and remove the stones, keeping the skin intact. Cut the flesh into quarters. *3* Add all the ingredients except the Swiss chard to the blender and secure the lid. *4* Starting at low speed and gradually increasing toward high, blend the ingredients for 1 minute or until the mixture contains no visible pieces of fruit. *5* Remove and discard the stems of the Swiss chard. Add the Swiss chard and blend again at medium speed for 30 seconds, gradually increasing the speed to high. Blend on high speed for another 15 to 30 seconds or until the entire mixture is smooth. *6* Pour the smoothie into two glasses and enjoy!

Per serving: Calories 211 (From Fat 54); Fat 6g (Saturated 1g); Cholesterol 0mg; Sodium 55mg; Carbohydrate 38g (Dietary Fiber 10g); Protein 6g.

Tip: If you don't have fresh ginger, use ¼ teaspoon of ground ginger instead. If you don't have chia seeds, use 1 tablespoon of ground flaxseed instead. If you don't have access to peaches, try 2 peeled kiwis.

Cucumber and Melon Natural Slender

Prep time: 3–4 min • **Blending time:** 2 min • **Yield:** 2 servings

Ingredients	Directions
1 cucumber, peeled and chopped 2 cups chopped honeydew 2 tablespoons fresh lime juice 1 tablespoon psyllium husk powder ½ cup coconut water 1½ cups water 2 cups dandelion leaves, loosely packed	*1* Combine all the ingredients except the dandelion leaves in the blender and secure the lid. *2* Starting at low speed and gradually increasing toward high, blend the ingredients for 30 to 45 seconds or until the mixture contains no visible pieces of fruit. *3* Add the dandelion leaves and blend again at medium speed for 30 seconds, gradually increasing the speed to high. Blend on high speed for another 15 to 30 seconds or until the entire mixture is smooth. *4* Pour the smoothie into two glasses and enjoy!

Per serving: Calories 123 (From Fat 9); Fat 1g (Saturated 0g); Cholesterol 0mg; Sodium 143mg; Carbohydrate 29g (Dietary Fiber 7g); Protein 3g.

Tip: If you don't have honeydew melon, use 2 cups of chopped fresh cantaloupe instead. If you don't have fresh dandelion leaves at your local farmers' market, choose mustard greens, beet greens, or parsnip greens instead.

Vary It! Add 3 or 4 mint leaves for a fresh flavor.

Dazzling Passion Fruit, Papaya, and Cinnamon

Prep time: 3–4 min • **Blending time:** 2 min • **Yield:** 2 servings

Ingredients	Directions
2 passion fruits	*1* Cut the passion fruits in half and scoop out the seeded pulp from the center. Keep the pulp and discard the shells.
3 cups chopped papaya, seeded and peeled	
1 tablespoon ground flaxseed	*2* Combine all the ingredients except the watercress in the blender and secure the lid.
¼ teaspoon ground cinnamon	
2 tablespoons fresh lime juice	*3* Starting at low speed and gradually increasing toward high, blend the ingredients for 45 seconds or until the mixture contains no visible pieces of fruit.
2 cups water	
2 cups watercress, loosely packed	
	4 Add the watercress and blend again at medium speed for 30 seconds, gradually increasing the speed to high. Blend on high speed for another 15 to 30 seconds or until the entire mixture is smooth.
	5 Pour the smoothie into two glasses and enjoy!

Per serving: Calories 131 (From Fat 18); Fat 2g (Saturated 0g); Cholesterol 0mg; Sodium 43mg; Carbohydrate 30g (Dietary Fiber 7g); Protein 3g.

Tip: If you don't have access to fresh papaya, use 2 cups of fresh pineapple and half a cucumber instead.

Watermelon Kiwi Lime Creation

Prep time: 25 min • **Blending time:** 2 min • **Yield:** 2 servings

Ingredients	Directions
2 tablespoons chia seeds	*1* Place the chia seeds in a bowl with ¼ cup of room temperature water. Place in the fridge to soak for at least 20 minutes or overnight.
3 cups chopped watermelon	
2 kiwis, peeled	
¼ cup fresh lime juice	*2* Combine the chia seeds, watermelon, kiwis, lime juice, and water in the blender and secure the lid.
1 cup water	
1 cup celery leaves, loosely packed	
3 romaine lettuce leaves	*3* Starting at low speed and gradually increasing toward high, blend the ingredients for 45 seconds or until the mixture contains no visible pieces of fruit.
	4 Add the celery leaves and lettuce and blend again at medium speed for 30 seconds, gradually increasing the speed to high. Blend on high speed for another 15 to 30 seconds or until the entire mixture is smooth.
	5 Pour the smoothie into two glasses and enjoy!

Per serving: Calories 249 (From Fat 72); Fat 8g (Saturated 1g); Cholesterol 0mg; Sodium 52mg; Carbohydrate 44g (Dietary Fiber 12g); Protein 7g.

Tip: If you want a sweeter taste without added calories, add 1 teaspoon of stevia powder.

Vary It! In winter months, you can use 3 cups of red or green grapes instead of watermelon.

Chapter 13

Green Smoothies for Chronic or Serious Medical Conditions

*I*f you or someone you love has suffered from a major health problem like heart disease, diabetes, or cancer, you know firsthand how quickly sickness can change the quality of life.

Sickness is a real part of life, but it doesn't have to take over your life. Using natural foods to help you rebalance, rebuild, repair, and heal can help your body recover better and more quickly. And the sooner you can get better, the sooner you can get back to enjoying a healthy life again.

My genuine wish for you is that you're not sick yet and are actively taking steps toward prevention by reading this book. In that case, you can use the recipes in this chapter to strengthen your body, immune system, and overall health. If you have a family history of one particular type of ailment, such as heart disease or arthritis, focus on the recipes in that corresponding section to strengthen your own natural defenses in that area.

If you're already suffering from some type of illness, then you've come to the right place. In this chapter, I outline some of the most common ailments and diseases affecting people today. I highlight specific foods to help combat illness naturally and strengthen the body back to health, and I provide smoothie recipes targeted to those ailments. This chapter is all about teaching you how foods can help you both prevent disease and manage disease for a happier, healthier you.

> *Recipes in This Chapter (cont.)*
>
> ▶ Basil and Sunflower Sprouts Sensation
>
> ▶ Hemp, Orange, and Chia Medley
>
> ▶ Revitalizing Pineapple, Cilantro, and Lime
>
> ▶ Soothing Celery, Fennel, and Cucumber
>
> ▶ Raspberry, Clementine, and Chlorella Power
>
>

Winning the Battle with Inflammation

What do swollen and painful joints, arthritis, injuries that won't heal, inflammatory bowel disease (IBD), autoimmune disease, allergies, asthma, puffiness in the arms and face, and even higher risk for certain types of cancer all have in common? All these health issues revolve around one main condition: chronic inflammation.

You can understand how normal levels of inflammation work whenever you stub your toe or bump your head. You probably notice the swelling and inflammation pretty quickly as your immune system sends more blood to the wound to start the process of healing. When the job is finished, your immune system goes back to other important tasks, and the inflammation goes away.

Normal amounts of inflammation turn *chronic* when the immune system keeps trying to fix a persistent problem, constantly sending more blood throughout the body and putting the inflammation into overdrive. Chronic inflammation is a leading factor in chronic disease. Reducing inflammation prevents many types of disease and promotes faster healing if you do get sick.

Factors that cause or contribute to chronic inflammation include the following:

✔ Poor diet, including refined sugar, refined flours, and processed foods

✔ Chronic infections from viruses, bacteria, yeast, or parasites

> ✔ Hidden allergens from food or the environment
>
> ✔ Underlying autoimmune conditions

Of all these factors, the one you can control the most is diet. Eating a diet rich in fresh fruits and vegetables helps minimize inflammation in the first place. Here are some other ways to make over your diet:

✔ Transition away from inflammatory foods such as alcohol, refined sugar, and processed carbs (such as pasta, chips, crackers, cookies, and white bread).

✔ Break the habit of consuming acidic foods like coffee and sugary sodas.

✔ Avoid bad fats in fried foods and keep animal-based fats to a minimum.

✔ Increase your intake of foods that are anti-inflammatory, such as guava, bell pepper, citrus fruits, berries, lemons, kiwi, pomegranate, and leafy greens. Turmeric, fennel, cinnamon, nutmeg, ginger, and manuka honey are especially known to have excellent anti-inflammatory effects.

Add high antioxidant superfoods like acai powder, goji berries, or pomegranate powder to any of the recipes in this section for even more anti-inflammatory effects. Chapter 6 provides a detailed explanation of superfoods and how to use them in your smoothies.

Check out *Anti-Inflammation Diet For Dummies* by Dr. Artemis Morris and Molly Rossiter (Wiley) for more information on inflammation and recipes to help you combat it.

Avoiding monosodium glutamate (MSG)

Monosodium glutamate (MSG) is a salty flavor enhancer that adds a savory taste to food. Manufacturers often use it as an inexpensive flavor booster in soup stocks, chips and crackers, sauces, salad dressings, frozen dinners, airplane food, and fast food.

MSG is a known cause of inflammation, but it often falls under the radar because of the widespread lack of knowledge of its potential health effects. The United States Food and Drug Administration granted MSG a Generally Recognized as Safe (GRAS) status back in 1958, and no one's looked at it again since, essentially giving the food industry a free pass to use as much of it as it wants in your food.

To keep your diet free of MSG, check the ingredient labels on your foods, especially salty, savory products. MSG may be listed as MSG, 621, or E621, or it may not be listed at all. MSG can hide in other ingredients like "natural flavorings" and "spices." In these cases, food companies can still label a food as having "no added MSG," so if you see either of those ingredients listed, your best bet is to avoid that product.

Dill-ightful Ginger and Turmeric

Prep time: 3–4 min • **Blending time:** 2 min • **Yield:** 2 servings

Ingredients	*Directions*
½ avocado, peeled and pitted	**1** Combine the avocado, cucumber, ginger, turmeric, lime juice, and water in the blender and secure the lid.
1 cucumber, peeled and chopped	
½-inch piece fresh ginger (peeled)	**2** Starting at low speed and gradually increasing toward high, blend the ingredients for 30 to 45 seconds or until the mixture contains no visible pieces of ingredients.
½ teaspoon ground turmeric	
½ cup fresh lime juice	**3** Add the dill, celery leaves, and mustard greens and blend again at medium speed for 30 seconds, gradually increasing the speed to high. Blend on high speed for another 15 to 30 seconds or until the entire mixture is smooth.
1 cup water	
¼ cup fresh dill, loosely packed	
1 cup celery leaves, loosely packed	
1 cup baby mustard greens, loosely packed	**4** Pour the smoothie into two glasses and enjoy!

Per serving: Calories 131 (From Fat 54); Fat 6g (Saturated 1g); Cholesterol 0mg; Sodium 63mg; Carbohydrate 19g (Dietary Fiber 5g); Protein 4g.

Tip: If you don't have fresh dill, use ¼ cup of fresh cilantro instead. If you don't have fresh ginger, use ¼ teaspoon of ground ginger instead.

Tip: Add a pinch of Himalayan salt to bring out more of the savory flavors. Add a dash of cayenne pepper for a spicy kick.

Vary It! Replace the cucumber with a tomato for a slightly different taste.

Refreshing Kiwi and Cilantro

Prep time: 3–4 min • **Blending time:** 2 min • **Yield:** 2 servings

Ingredients	Directions
1 red delicious or gala apple	*1* Cut the apple and remove the core, keeping the skin intact. Cut the flesh into quarters.
2 kiwis, peeled	
½-inch piece fresh ginger (peeled)	*2* Add the apple, kiwis, ginger, flaxseed, and water to the blender and secure the lid.
2 tablespoons ground flaxseed	
1½ cups water	*3* Starting at low speed and gradually increasing toward high, blend the ingredients for 1 minute or until the mixture contains no visible pieces of fruit.
1 cup cilantro, loosely packed	
1 cup baby spinach, loosely packed	
	4 Add the cilantro and spinach and blend again at medium speed for 45 seconds, gradually increasing the speed to high. Blend on high speed for another 15 to 30 seconds or until the entire mixture is smooth.
	5 Pour the smoothie into two glasses.

Per serving: Calories 159 (From Fat 27); Fat 3g (Saturated 0g); Cholesterol 0mg; Sodium 28mg; Carbohydrate 32g (Dietary Fiber 6g); Protein 4g.

Tip: If you don't have fresh ginger, use ¼ teaspoon of ground ginger instead.

Vary It! Replace the apple with 1 cup of fresh pineapple chunks for a sweeter smoothie.

Hearty Kale, Blueberry, and Hemp

Prep time: 3–4 min • **Blending time:** 2 min • **Yield:** 2 servings

Ingredients	Directions
½ avocado, peeled and pitted	*1* Combine all the ingredients except the kale in the blender and secure the lid.
1½ cups blueberries	
1 tablespoon raw almond butter	*2* Starting at low speed and gradually increasing toward high, blend the ingredients for 30 to 45 seconds or until smooth and the mixture contains no visible pieces of fruit.
2 tablespoons ground hemp seeds	
2 tablespoons manuka honey	
1½ cups water	*3* Remove and discard the stems of the kale. Add the kale and blend again at medium speed for 30 seconds, gradually increasing the speed to high. Blend on high speed for another 15 to 30 seconds or until the entire mixture is smooth.
4 large kale leaves	
	4 Pour the smoothie into two glasses and enjoy!

Per serving: Calories 290 (From Fat 153); Fat 17g (Saturated 1.5g); Cholesterol 0mg; Sodium 22mg; Carbohydrate 31g (Dietary Fiber 6g); Protein 9g.

Tip: If you can't find fresh blueberries, use store-bought frozen ones instead. Just check the ingredients label to make sure they contain no added sugar. If you don't have raw almond butter, use 3 or 4 raw almonds instead.

Nutmeg, Cinnamon, and Celery Surprise

Prep time: 3–4 min • **Blending time:** 2 min • **Yield:** 2 servings

Ingredients	Directions
2 guavas	*1* Cut the guavas, keeping the skin intact, and remove any large seeds (small seeds are okay). Cut the flesh into quarters.
1 ripe banana, peeled	
¼ teaspoon ground nutmeg	
½ teaspoon ground cinnamon	*2* Add the guava, banana, nutmeg, cinnamon, flaxseed, and water to the blender and secure the lid.
2 tablespoons ground flaxseed	
1½ cups water	*3* Starting at low speed and gradually increasing toward high, blend the ingredients for 1 minute or until the mixture contains no visible pieces of fruit.
1 cup baby spinach, loosely packed	
1 cup celery leaves, loosely packed	*4* Add the spinach and celery leaves and blend again at medium speed for 45 seconds, gradually increasing the speed to high. Blend on high speed for another 15 to 30 seconds or until the entire mixture is smooth.
	5 Pour the smoothie into two glasses and enjoy.

Per serving: Calories 134 (From Fat 27); Fat 3g (Saturated 0.5g); Cholesterol 0mg; Sodium 58mg; Carbohydrate 26g (Dietary Fiber 8g); Protein 4g.

Tip: If you don't have fresh guava, use an apple or a pear instead.

Vary It! For a slightly different taste, add a pinch of ground cloves, ground cardamom, or 1 to 2 teaspoons of vanilla extract.

Pomegranate, Fennel, and Tangerine Dream

Prep time: 25 min • **Blending time:** 2 min • **Yield:** 2 servings

Ingredients	Directions
2 tablespoons chia seeds **1 cup fresh pomegranate seeds**	**1** Place the chia seeds in a bowl with ¼ cup of room temperature water. Place in the fridge to soak for at least 20 minutes or overnight.
4 tangerines, peeled and seeded **2 tablespoons fresh lemon juice**	**2** Combine the chia seeds, pomegranate seeds, tangerine, lemon juice, orange oil, and water in the blender and secure the lid.
1 drop pure wild orange essential oil **1½ cups water**	**3** Starting at low speed and gradually increasing toward high, blend the ingredients for 1 minute or until the mixture contains no visible pieces of fruit.
¼ cup chopped fennel, loosely packed **2 cups watercress, loosely packed**	**4** Add the fennel and watercress and blend again at medium speed for 30 seconds, gradually increasing the speed to high. Blend on high speed for another 15 to 30 seconds or until the entire mixture is smooth.
	5 Pour the smoothie into two glasses and enjoy!

Per serving: Calories 294 (From Fat 63); Fat 7g (Saturated 1g); Cholesterol 0mg; Sodium 35mg; Carbohydrate 58g (Dietary Fiber 15g); Protein 7g.

Tip: If you don't have time to soak your chia seeds for the full 20 minutes, try adding them to the 1½ cups water while you prepare the other ingredients. When you're ready to add the water, add the chia seeds and water together.

Tip: Use 2 oranges (peeled and seeded) if you don't have tangerines. If fresh fennel isn't available, use ¼ teaspoon of ground fennel instead.

Lemon, Lime, and Parsley Twist

Prep time: 4–5 min • **Blending time:** 2 min • **Yield:** 2 servings

Ingredients	Directions
½ **red bell pepper, seeded and quartered**	*1* Combine the bell pepper, avocado, cucumber, lemon juice, lime juice, vinegar, cayenne, and water in the blender and secure the lid.
½ **avocado, peeled and pitted**	
1 cucumber, peeled and chopped	
2 tablespoons fresh lemon juice	*2* Starting at low speed and gradually increasing toward high, blend the ingredients for 30 to 45 seconds or until the mixture contains no visible pieces of ingredients.
2 tablespoons fresh lime juice	
2 tablespoons raw apple cider vinegar	
Dash of cayenne pepper to taste	*3* Add the parsley and cilantro and blend again at medium speed for 30 seconds, gradually increasing the speed to high. Blend on high speed for another 15 to 30 seconds or until the entire mixture is smooth.
1 cup water	
1½ **cups parsley, loosely packed**	
½ **cup cilantro, loosely packed**	*4* Pour the smoothie into two glasses and enjoy!

Per serving: Calories 132 (From Fat 54); Fat 6g (Saturated 1g); Cholesterol 0mg; Sodium 52mg; Carbohydrate 19g (Dietary Fiber 6g); Protein 5g.

Tip: You can also use fresh hot pepper instead of cayenne, but use a small amount. Depending on how many seeds you include, just ⅛ teaspoon of chopped fresh jalapeño or habanero pepper can add a lot of kick!

Bring on the peppers but hold the hot sauce!

Although fresh hot peppers invoke the feeling of a hot, flaming fire, they're actually a very beneficial anti-inflammatory food. The anti-inflammatory effect comes directly from *capsaicin,* the compound found primarily in the hot pepper's seeds, which is proven to block pro-inflammatory chain reactions in the blood. However, not all heat is created equal. Though peppers reduce inflammation, hot pepper sauces often contain added sugar and/or MSG, which both *promote* inflammation. Your best bet: Choose fresh hot peppers or stick with ground cayenne.

Minimizing Heart Disease Risk

The biggest cause of death today is heart disease. More than 600,000 Americans die every year from heart disease, making it the leading cause of death of men and women in the United States. What's worse, the numbers just keep rising every year.

Heart disease, or cardiovascular disease, most commonly occurs from a condition called atherosclerosis. *Atherosclerosis* develops when plaque builds up in the walls of the arteries. This buildup narrows the arteries and restricts blood flow. If even a small blood clot forms, it can stop the blood flow and trigger a heart attack or stroke.

High blood pressure, high cholesterol, and smoking are key risk factors for heart disease. According to the Centers for Disease Control and Prevention (CDC), about half of all Americans have at least one of these three risk factors. Several other medical conditions and lifestyle choices can also increase your risk for heart disease, including

- Diabetes
- Excess weight and obesity
- Poor diet
- Physical inactivity
- Excessive alcohol use

Taking active steps to prevent heart disease is really critical because the first symptom of heart disease is often death. That's why it's called "the silent killer."

To reduce your risk of heart disease, eat a healthy diet that's low in salt, low in animal-based fats, and high in fresh fruits and vegetables. Choose foods that help strengthen your heart and increase circulation, including dark leafy bitter greens (think green smoothie), cayenne pepper, ginger, turmeric, cinnamon, raw apple cider vinegar, oranges, avocados, almonds, walnuts, flaxseeds, and berries. Exercise on a regular basis, try to keep your stress levels low, and avoid smoking.

Almond Blueberri-licious

Prep time: 3–4 min • **Blending time:** 2 min • **Yield:** 2 servings

Ingredients	Directions
¼ **cup raw almonds** **2 cups water**	***1*** Combine the almonds and water in the blender and secure the lid.
2 ripe bananas, peeled **1 cup blueberries** ½ **cup raspberries**	***2*** Starting at low speed and gradually increasing toward high, blend the ingredients for 30 to 45 seconds or until the mixture is smooth.
2 tablespoons ground flaxseed **4 mint leaves** **3 large Swiss chard leaves**	***3*** Add the bananas, blueberries, raspberries, and flaxseed and blend again at medium speed for 45 seconds, gradually increasing the speed to high.
	4 Remove and discard the stems of the Swiss chard. Add the Swiss chard and mint and blend again at medium speed for 30 seconds, gradually increasing the speed to high. Blend on high speed for another 15 to 30 seconds or until the entire mixture is smooth.
	5 Pour the smoothie into two glasses and enjoy!

Per serving: Calories 303 (From Fat 117); Fat 13g (Saturated 1g); Cholesterol 0mg; Sodium 51mg; Carbohydrate 47g (Dietary Fiber 11g); Protein 8g.

Tip: You can use a drop of pure peppermint oil instead of fresh mint leaves.

Vary It! Use blackberries or strawberries instead of blueberries or raspberries.

Delightful Orange Cinnamon

Prep time: 3–4 min • **Blending time:** 2 min • **Yield:** 2 servings

Ingredients	Directions
1 orange, peeled and seeded	*1* Combine all the ingredients except the lettuce in the blender and secure the lid.
½ avocado, peeled and pitted	
1 Medjool date, pitted	*2* Starting at low speed and gradually increasing toward high, blend the ingredients for 30 to 45 seconds or until the mixture contains are no visible pieces of fruit.
2 tablespoons ground flaxseed	
½ teaspoon ground cinnamon	
1½ cups water	*3* Add the lettuce and blend again at medium speed for 30 seconds, gradually increasing the speed to high. Blend on high speed for another 15 to 30 seconds or until the entire mixture is smooth.
4 large romaine lettuce leaves	
	4 Pour the smoothie into two glasses and enjoy!

Per serving: Calories 155 (From Fat 72); Fat 8g (Saturated 1g); Cholesterol 0mg; Sodium 10mg; Carbohydrate 23g (Dietary Fiber 7g); Protein 3g.

Tip: If you don't have Medjool dates, use 1 tablespoon of raw honey instead.

Vary It! Add a dash of cayenne pepper instead of cinnamon. For an even sweeter flavor, replace the orange with 2 tangerines.

Sweet Walnut Ginger Apple

Prep time: 3–4 min • **Blending time:** 2 min • **Yield:** 2 servings

Ingredients	Directions
2 red apples	*1* Cut the apples and remove the cores, keeping the skin intact. Cut the flesh into quarters.
1 ripe banana, peeled	
6 whole raw, unsalted walnuts or 10 walnut pieces	*2* Combine all the ingredients except the dandelion greens in the blender and secure the lid.
2 tablespoons raw apple cider vinegar	
1 tablespoon manuka honey	*3* Starting at low speed and gradually increasing toward high, blend the ingredients for 30 to 45 seconds or until the mixture contains no visible pieces of fruit.
½-inch piece fresh ginger (peeled)	
2 cups water	
2 cups fresh dandelion greens, loosely packed	*4* Cut away the stems of the dandelion greens. Add the dandelion greens and blend again at medium speed for 30 seconds, gradually increasing the speed to high. Blend on high speed for another 30 seconds or until the entire mixture is smooth.
	5 Pour the smoothie into two glasses and enjoy!

Per serving: Calories 310 (From Fat 81); Fat 9g (Saturated 1g); Cholesterol 0mg; Sodium 57mg; Carbohydrate 59g (Dietary Fiber 9g); Protein 5g.

Tip: Use baby spinach or baby kale leaves if you don't have dandelion greens. If you don't have fresh ginger, use ¼ teaspoon of ground ginger instead.

Vary It! Use ½ teaspoon of ground turmeric instead of or along with the ginger. For a spicy kick, add a dash of cayenne pepper. Add ½ teaspoon of ground cinnamon for a sweeter, dessert-like flavor.

Pineapple Turmeric Surprise

Prep time: 3–4 min • **Blending time:** 2 min • **Yield:** 2 servings

Ingredients	Directions
1½ cups pineapple chunks	**1** Combine all the ingredients except the kale in the blender and secure the lid.
1 ripe banana, peeled	
½ teaspoon ground turmeric	**2** Starting at low speed and gradually increasing toward high, blend the ingredients for 30 to 45 seconds or until the mixture contains no visible pieces of fruit.
½-inch piece fresh ginger (peeled)	
2 tablespoons ground flaxseed	
1 tablespoon coconut oil	**3** Remove and discard the stems of the kale. Add the kale and blend again at medium speed for 30 seconds, gradually increasing the speed to high. Blend on high speed for another 15 to 30 seconds or until the entire mixture is smooth.
1½ cups water	
5 baby kale leaves	
	4 Pour the smoothie into two glasses and enjoy!

Per serving: Calories 289 (From Fat 90); Fat 10g (Saturated 6g); Cholesterol 0mg; Sodium 39mg; Carbohydrate 49g (Dietary Fiber 6g); Protein 4g.

Tip: If you don't have fresh ginger, use ¼ teaspoon of ground ginger instead.

Vary It! Instead of pineapple, add ½ cup of fresh mango or 2 kiwis, peeled and quartered. Or, for a sweet and spicy twist, try adding a small dash of cayenne pepper and a pinch of Himalayan salt.

Cha-Cha Chia Fruity Blend

Prep time: 25 min • **Blending time:** 2 min • **Yield:** 2 servings

Ingredients	Directions
2 tablespoons chia seeds, soaked for 20 minutes	**1** Place the chia seeds in a bowl with ¼ cup of room temperature water. Place in the fridge to soak for at least 20 minutes or overnight.
1 ripe pear	
½ avocado, peeled and pitted	
1 orange, peeled and seeded	**2** Cut the pear and remove the core, keeping the skin intact. Cut the flesh into quarters.
1½ cups halved strawberries, stems and leaves removed	
2½ cups water	**3** Combine all the ingredients except the spinach in the blender and secure the lid.
2 cups baby spinach, loosely packed	**4** Starting at low speed and gradually increasing toward high, blend the ingredients for 30 to 45 seconds or until the mixture contains no visible pieces of fruit.
	5 Add the spinach and blend again at medium speed for 30 seconds, gradually increasing the speed to high. Blend on high speed for another 15 to 30 seconds or until the entire mixture is smooth.
	6 Pour the smoothie into two glasses and enjoy!

Per serving: Calories 248 (From Fat 90); Fat 10g (Saturated 1g); Cholesterol 0mg; Sodium 38mg; Carbohydrate 39g (Dietary Fiber 14g); Protein 5g.

Tip: Use 2 cups of freshly pressed orange juice instead of water for a really fruity taste!

Vary It! Try replacing the spinach with different greens, such as bok choy, mustard greens, or collard greens.

Navigating Diet Choices When You Have Diabetes

When I was a kid, diabetes was a rare disease that you only heard about occasionally. Today, diabetes is the world's fastest-growing chronic condition, and those being diagnosed are younger and younger. At least 1 in 8 people with diabetes is now under the age of 40, compared with about 1 in 30 people just 20 years ago. Diabetes remains the leading cause of kidney failure and blindness in older adults and is the cause of thousands of amputations a year. It's also a major contributor to heart disease and stroke. If left untreated, diabetes can be life threatening.

When I say "diabetes," I'm talking primarily about *Type 2 diabetes,* which is often caused by lifestyle and accounts for 90 to 95 percent of all diagnosed cases. *Type 1 diabetes* is an autoimmune condition and usually starts in childhood or early youth. Exactly what causes Type 1 diabetes is still somewhat mysterious, although most people seem to agree that genetic or environmental factors may be involved.

Gestational diabetes is another form of glucose intolerance that can affect some women during pregnancy. After pregnancy, about 5 to 10 percent of women who have gestational diabetes develop Type 2 diabetes.

Don't think that you can't have any green smoothies as a diabetic. The recipes in this section show you how to use the right foods for your condition. For example, stevia powder provides a sweet taste without the added sugar content. Dark leafy green vegetables contain virtually no sugar, so they're a great food choice for diabetics. Cucumber, bell pepper, avocado, celery, lemon, lime, ginger, turmeric, flaxseeds, chia seeds, and almonds are all good smoothie ingredients because they help balance blood sugars. Fruits that are naturally low in sugar, such as grapefruit, blueberries, and blackberries, are also suitable choices.

Sweet Stevia and Sour Green Apple

Prep time: 3–4 min • **Blending time:** 2 min • **Yield:** 2 servings

Ingredients	Directions
½ **green apple**	*1* Cut the apple and remove the core, keeping the skin intact.
1 cucumber, peeled and chopped	
¼ **teaspoon ground cinnamon**	*2* Combine the apple, cucumber, cinnamon, flaxseed, stevia powder, and water in the blender and secure the lid.
2 tablespoons ground flaxseed	
1 teaspoon stevia powder	*3* Starting at low speed and gradually increasing toward high, blend the ingredients for 30 to 45 seconds or until the mixture contains no visible pieces of fruit.
1 cup water	
1½ cups celery leaves, loosely packed	
½ **cup mint leaves, loosely packed**	*4* Add the celery and mint and blend again at medium speed for 30 seconds, gradually increasing the speed to high. Blend on high speed for another 30 seconds or until the entire mixture is smooth.
	5 Pour the smoothie into two glasses and enjoy!

Per serving: Calories 83 (From Fat 23); Fat 2.5g (Saturated 0g); Cholesterol 0mg; Sodium 68mg; Carbohydrate 17g (Dietary Fiber 5g); Protein 3g.

Vary It! Try using a cup of chopped fresh fennel instead of celery. You can also add a dash of raw apple cider vinegar or a tablespoon of lemon juice.

Fresh Parsley, Goji, and Grapefruit

Prep time: 25 min • **Blending time:** 2 min • **Yield:** 2 servings

Ingredients	Directions
2 tablespoons goji berries ½ grapefruit, peeled and seeded 2 tablespoons ground flaxseed 1 tablespoon coconut oil 1½ cups water 1 cup parsley, loosely packed ½ cup baby spinach, loosely packed	*1* Place the goji berries in a bowl with ¼ cup of room temperature water. Place in the fridge to soak for at least 20 minutes or overnight. *2* Combine the goji berries, grapefruit, flaxseed, coconut oil, and water in the blender and secure the lid. *3* Starting at low speed and gradually increasing toward high, blend the ingredients for 1 minute or until the mixture contains no visible pieces of fruit. *4* Add the parsley and spinach and blend again at medium speed for 30 seconds, gradually increasing the speed to high. Blend on high speed for another 15 to 30 seconds or until the entire mixture is smooth. *5* Pour the smoothie into two glasses and enjoy!

Per serving: Calories 202 (From Fat 81); Fat 9g (Saturated 6g); Cholesterol 0mg; Sodium 28mg; Carbohydrate 27g (Dietary Fiber 4g); Protein 6g.

Vary It! Add ½-inch piece of peeled fresh ginger or ¼ teaspoon of ground ginger for a slightly different taste.

Lemon Berry Avocado Nirvana

Prep time: 3–4 min • **Blending time:** 2 min • **Yield:** 2 servings

Ingredients	Directions
½ **avocado, peeled and pitted** **2 tablespoons fresh lemon juice** ½ **cup raspberries** ½ **cup blueberries** 1½ **cups water** **4 mint leaves** **3 Swiss chard leaves**	*1* Add the avocado, lemon juice, raspberries, blueberries, and water to the blender and secure the lid. *2* Starting at low speed and gradually increasing toward high, blend the ingredients for 1 minute or until the mixture contains no visible pieces of fruit. *3* Remove and discard the stems of the Swiss chard. Add the mint and Swiss chard and blend again at medium speed for 30 to 45 seconds, gradually increasing the speed to high. Blend on high speed for another 15 to 30 seconds or until the entire mixture is smooth. *4* Pour the smoothie into two glasses and enjoy!

Per serving: Calories 99 (From Fat 54); Fat 6g (Saturated 1g); Cholesterol 0mg; Sodium 47mg; Carbohydrate 14g (Dietary Fiber 5g); Protein 2g.

Tip: If Swiss chard tastes too bitter for you, try using 2 cups of baby spinach instead. Add ½ teaspoon of stevia powder for a sweeter taste.

Using the glycemic index (GI) with foods

The *glycemic index (GI)* is a scientific measure of how your blood sugar reacts to eating a particular food. Think of it as a simple good carbs/bad carbs measure to understand how certain carbohydrates affect your blood sugar. The GI ranks foods from a score of 0 to 110. Foods with an index of 55 or lower are considered low-GI foods; those with an index of 56 to 69 are medium; and those scored 70 or higher are considered high-GI. As a diabetic, using the GI can help you determine which foods are okay to eat and which foods are best to avoid. Highly refined foods such as donuts, cookies, pies, white bread, and potato chips have a high GI score and cause a blood sugar spike. Choosing low-GI foods such as beans, legumes, non-starchy veggies, most fruits, and many whole-grain breads and cereals results in a much lower impact on blood glucose levels.

Vanilla, Coconut, and Almond Fusion

Prep time: 4–5 min • **Blending time:** 2 min • **Yield:** 2 servings

Ingredients	Directions
½ ripe banana, peeled	*1* Combine all the ingredients except the spinach in the blender and secure the lid.
½ cup blueberries	
1 tablespoon coconut oil	*2* Starting at low speed and gradually easing toward high, blend the ingredients for 1 minute or until smooth.
1 teaspoon stevia powder	
2 tablespoons raw almond butter	
½ tablespoon raw cacao powder	*3* Add the spinach and blend again at medium speed for 45 seconds, gradually increasing the speed to high. Blend on high speed for another 15 to 30 seconds or until the entire mixture is smooth.
¼ teaspoon vanilla extract	
1½ cups water	
2 cups baby spinach	*4* Pour the smoothie into two glasses and enjoy!

Per serving: Calories 218 (From Fat 144); Fat 16g (Saturated 7g); Cholesterol 0mg; Sodium 30mg; Carbohydrate 20g (Dietary Fiber 4g); Protein 5g.

Tip: If you don't have raw almond butter, use 5 or 6 raw almonds instead.

Vary It! Try adding ¼ teaspoon of ground turmeric. If the taste of turmeric is too strong for you, use ¼ teaspoon of ground ginger instead. Add ½ cup of fresh raspberries instead of banana.

Basil and Sunflower Sprouts Sensation

Prep time: 4–5 min • **Blending time:** 2 min • **Yield:** 2 servings

Ingredients	Directions
½ **avocado, peeled and pitted**	*1* Add the avocado, bell pepper, onion, lime juice, cumin, and water to the blender and secure the lid.
½ **yellow bell pepper, seeded and quartered**	
½ **tablespoon minced white onion**	*2* Starting at low speed and gradually increasing toward high, blend the ingredients for 1 minute or until the mixture contains no visible pieces of ingredients.
1 tablespoon fresh lime juice	
¼ **teaspoon ground cumin**	
1½ **cups water**	*3* Add the sunflower sprouts and basil and blend again at medium speed for 30 to 45 seconds, gradually increasing the speed to high. Blend on high speed for another 15 to 30 seconds or until the entire mixture is smooth.
½ **cup sunflower sprouts, loosely packed**	
3 basil leaves	
1 cup baby spinach, loosely packed	
	4 Pour the smoothie into two glasses and enjoy!

Per serving: Calories 77 (From Fat 45); Fat 5g (Saturated 1g); Cholesterol 0mg; Sodium 41mg; Carbohydrate 8g (Dietary Fiber 3g); Protein 2g.

Tip: Add a dash of Himalayan sea salt for added flavor. If you don't like cumin, use a dash of cayenne pepper (to taste) instead.

Vary It! Replace the sunflower sprouts with ½ cup of fresh celery leaves.

Hemp, Orange, and Chia Medley

Prep time: 25 min • **Blending time:** 2 min • **Yield:** 2 servings

Ingredients	Directions
2 tablespoons chia seeds	**1** Place the chia seeds in a bowl with ¼ cup of room temperature water. Place in the fridge to soak for at least 20 minutes or overnight.
½ avocado, peeled and pitted	
½ cup raspberries	
½ ripe banana, peeled	**2** Add all the ingredients except the kale to the blender and secure the lid.
2 tablespoons ground hemp seed	
1 teaspoon stevia powder	**3** Starting at low speed and gradually increasing toward high, blend the ingredients for 1 minute or until the mixture contains no visible pieces of fruit.
2 drops pure wild orange essential oil	
1½ cups water	
4 large kale leaves	**4** Remove and discard the stems of the kale. Add the kale and blend again at medium speed for 30 seconds, gradually increasing the speed to high. Blend on high speed for another 15 to 30 seconds or until the entire mixture is smooth.
	5 Pour the smoothie into two glasses and enjoy!

Per serving: Calories 271 (From Fat 153); Fat 17g (Saturated 2g); Cholesterol 0mg; Sodium 24mg; Carbohydrate 27g (Dietary Fiber 12g); Protein 10g.

Note: The wild orange essential oil in this smoothie gives you the yummy natural flavor of oranges without the added sugar!

Vary It! You can switch up the flavor of this smoothie by replacing the orange oil with other 100 percent pure essential oils. Try 1 or 2 drops of peppermint, grapefruit, or lemon oil instead.

Healing after Surgery, Chemo, or Radiation

Any type of injury or illness can compromise your immune system and leave you feeling weak, lethargic, and basically wiped out. Your body can recover, but you need to support it through the process with the right foods, plenty of rest, and minimal stress. And of course, lots of love helps, too!

Healing after surgery takes time. The anesthesia alone can make you feel disoriented and weak. You may experience pain and notice more swelling in the first few days. If you've had surgery, remember that many side effects go away within a few days of the operation. With chemotherapy or radiation, your entire body is affected by the treatment, and your entire body needs to recover.

After surgery or treatment, your healing diet should focus on

- ✔ Minimizing and fighting inflammation with anti-inflammatory foods such as fresh ginger, turmeric, fennel, and all dark leafy greens (and without refined sugar, alcohol, processed foods, fried foods, meat, dairy, and wheat)

- ✔ Repairing your cells, boosting your immune system, and supporting your liver with foods high in antioxidants

- ✔ Detoxifying from the effects of chemo or radiation with foods such as cilantro and chlorella

- ✔ Encouraging bone and tissue healing with chlorophyll, found in dark leafy greens

- ✔ Hydrating your body with fluids

These recommended foods are all great smoothie ingredients. Making a green smoothie requires minimal effort and offers maximum support for your healing.

No matter what you're healing from, understand that the amount of time needed to recover is different for each person. Give your body the time it needs to rest. Combining rest with a healing diet can help you make a full recovery, get your immune system back to the top of its game again, and enjoy a healthy, happy life.

For another bonus recipe for a smoothie when you're recovering from surgery, chemo, or radiation, go to www.dummies.com/extras/greensmoothies to know how to make the Acai, Pomegranate, and Goji Berry green smoothie.

Revitalizing Pineapple, Cilantro, and Lime

Prep time: 3–4 min • **Blending time:** 2 min • **Yield:** 2 servings

Ingredients	Directions
¼ avocado, peeled and pitted	**1** Combine all the ingredients except the cilantro in the blender and secure the lid.
½ cucumber, peeled and chopped	
2 cups pineapple chunks	**2** Starting at low speed and gradually increasing toward high, blend the ingredients for 30 to 45 seconds or until the mixture contains no visible pieces of ingredients.
2 tablespoons fresh lime juice	
2 tablespoons ground flaxseed	
1½ cups water	**3** Add the cilantro and blend again at medium speed for 30 seconds, gradually increasing the speed to high. Blend on high speed for another 15 to 30 seconds or until the entire mixture is smooth.
2 cups cilantro, loosely packed	
	4 Pour the smoothie into two glasses and enjoy!

Per serving: Calories 242 (From Fat 72); Fat 8g (Saturated 1g); Cholesterol 0mg; Sodium 37mg; Carbohydrate 42g (Dietary Fiber 7g); Protein 3g.

Tip: Add a pinch of Himalayan salt for a natural flavor boost. Add ½ teaspoon of ground ginger or ground turmeric for more anti-inflammatory effects.

Combatting chemo side effects

Chemo actually brings on two types of side effects: the immediate ones, such as hair loss, nausea, loss of appetite, and dry mouth; and the lasting effects, such as *neuropathy* — tingling in the hands and feet — or hot flashes occurring from chemically induced menopause.

You may feel like your side effects are hanging around longer than you expected, or you may get lucky and have very few side effects at all. Be patient and set reasonable expectations. You may not be able to completely control how chemo affects your body, but you do have control over your diet and your mind. Focus your energy on putting only the very best foods in your body. Add the power of positive thinking, and you may find yourself feeling better more quickly and even minimizing any lingering effects. Every day after chemo is one day further on your recovery.

Soothing Celery, Fennel, and Cucumber

Prep time: 25 min • **Blending time:** 2 min • **Yield:** 2 servings

Ingredients	*Directions*
2 tablespoons chia seeds **1 cucumber, peeled and chopped** **½ cup chopped fennel** **2 tablespoons raw apple cider vinegar** **1 cup water** **4 mint leaves** **2 cups celery leaves, loosely packed**	*1* Place the chia seeds in a bowl with ¼ cup of room temperature water. Place in the fridge to soak for at least 20 minutes or overnight.
	2 Combine the chia seeds, cucumber, fennel, vinegar, and water in the blender and secure the lid.
	3 Starting at low speed and gradually increasing toward high, blend the ingredients for 1 minute or until the mixture contains no visible pieces of ingredients.
	4 Add the celery and mint and blend again at medium speed for 30 to 45 seconds, gradually increasing the speed to high. Blend on high speed for another 15 to 30 seconds or until the entire mixture is smooth.
	5 Pour the smoothie into two glasses and enjoy!

Per serving: Calories 113 (From Fat 45); Fat 5g (Saturated 0.5g); Cholesterol 0mg; Sodium 101mg; Carbohydrate 14g (Dietary Fiber 8g); Protein 4g.

Tip: If you can't find fresh fennel, use ½ teaspoon of ground fennel instead.

Vary It! Replace the mint with a dash of cayenne pepper for a more savory taste.

Raspberry, Clementine, and Chlorella Power

Prep time: 3–4 min • **Blending time:** 2 min • **Yield:** 2 servings

Ingredients	Directions
¼ avocado, peeled and pitted	*1* Combine all the ingredients except the kale in the blender and secure the lid.
4 clementines, peeled and seeded	
1 cup raspberries	*2* Starting at low speed and gradually increasing toward high, blend the ingredients for 30 to 45 seconds or until the mixture contains no visible pieces of fruit.
1 teaspoon chlorella powder	
1½ cups water	
4 large kale leaves	*3* Remove and discard the stems of the kale. Add the kale and blend again at medium speed for 30 seconds, gradually increasing the speed to high. Blend on high speed for another 15 to 30 seconds or until the entire mixture is smooth.
	4 Pour the smoothie into two glasses and enjoy!

Per serving: Calories 155 (From Fat 32); Fat 3.5g (Saturated 0g); Cholesterol 0mg; Sodium 21mg; Carbohydrate 30g (Dietary Fiber 8g); Protein 4g.

Tip: If you don't have raspberries, use fresh blueberries or blackberries instead.

Vary It! Add a dash of ground cinnamon for a heartier taste.

Chapter 14

Green Smoothies to Maximize Your Workouts

In This Chapter

▶ Benefitting from smoothies before and after workouts

▶ Using anti-inflammatory foods for muscle recovery and repair

Combining exercise with a healthy eating program gives you the absolute best chance of reaching an excellent state of health. Regular exercise keeps your heart healthy, your lungs strong, and your body fit. It can also help lower blood pressure and maintain steady blood sugar levels. Some studies even show that exercise helps improve sleep function, relieve symptoms of depression, increase self-esteem, and boost the immune system.

In order to tap into the health benefits of exercise, you have to give your body good fuel. For best results and long-term success, you need to eat nutrient-dense, easy-to-digest, fiber-rich, alkaline foods both before and after workouts. Hmmm . . . I think I know just the food!

A power-packed green smoothie before your workout gets you motivated to move your body and gives you the fuel you need to get a good workout and feel the burn. After you exercise, recharge and recover with green smoothies specially formulated to promote fast muscle recovery and keep that high energy feeling for the rest of the day. With the right foods, you'll find yourself hitting the gym, showing up for fitness class, or going for a run more than ever before.

Some recipes in this chapter call for bee pollen, which you should leave out if you're allergic to pollen or to bees. Even if you don't have one of these allergies, before including that ingredient in a smoothie flip to Chapter 6 for info on how to determine whether you're sensitive to consuming bee pollen.

Getting Nutrition before and after Workouts

If you eat before you exercise, your food needs to be light enough that it won't weigh you down or make you feel tired. For that, use high-water-content fruits such as apple, pineapple, grapes, kiwi, or cucumber and minimize fats like avocado or nuts. After a workout, a thicker, heartier smoothie helps curb your appetite, balance your blood sugar, and give you plenty of energy for hours after. A post-workout smoothie can have more healthy fats and should also have some natural anti-inflammatory foods (such as cinnamon or fresh fruit) to help your muscles recover and repair.

Benefitting from a pre-workout smoothie

Getting hydrated and mentally preparing yourself to get your body moving is important before exercise. If you eat heavy foods like pizza, pasta, or a large sub sandwich before trying to work out, your exercise will likely be limited to crawling to the sofa and collapsing into a carbohydrate coma. A green smoothie is easy on your digestion and naturally makes you feel energized. What better way to use that energy than to exercise! A pre-workout smoothie gives you the following:

- ✔ Higher energy levels for a better workout

- ✔ An easy-to-digest meal with no heartburn or indigestion

- ✔ Blended food in its natural form — nature's best fuel

- ✔ Plenty of magnesium, calcium, and potassium — nutrients that help maximize your body's performance

- ✔ Lots of hydration from the fruits, greens, and water

The best smoothies in this chapter to drink before workouts are Grape, Orange, and Spinach Motivator and Strawberry, Peach, and Maca Prep.

Recovering with a post-workout smoothie

After exercise, your metabolism works faster and is looking for good fuel (food). The worst thing you can do after a good workout is decelerate your metabolism with a big, heavy meal full of refined carbohydrates and empty calories. That kind of food diverts all your body's energy to digestion, so you don't have any energy left for recovery and repair (clearing lactic acid from the blood, removing other wastes, delivering nutrients, and so on). A green smoothie is already blended and therefore very easy for your body to digest. A post-workout smoothie gives you the following:

- Higher energy levels for the rest of the day
- Better muscle recovery/less lactic acid buildup
- More natural ability to balance blood sugars
- Fast and easy digestion and absorption
- Less hunger and reduced cravings for unhealthy foods
- Plenty of hydration to replenish electrolytes and fluids
- Natural anti-inflammatory effects that promote tissue repair and minimize injuries

The best smoothies in this chapter to drink after workouts are Banana, Spirulina, and Coconut Water Recharge; Chia, Raspberry, and Turmeric Zen; and High Power Tahini, Date, and Avocado.

Loading up on the best fuel

Your body needs three *macronutrients* (the nutrients required in the greatest amounts) on a daily basis: healthy carbohydrates, protein, and fat. (*Micronutrients* are the vitamins and minerals that your body also needs, but in much smaller amounts than the main macronutrients.) Each of these macronutrients supplies the body with energy. Carbohydrates are the most direct source of energy; you find them in the natural sugars in fruits. Good fats are what you get from nuts, seeds, cold-pressed oils, and avocados. (*Cold-pressed* oils are made by pressing the seeds, nuts, or fruits to release their oil.) Protein helps build stronger muscles and is found in all leafy greens, *spirulina* (a freshwater algae), nuts, seeds, and sprouts. Green smoothies are filled with all these macronutrients, blended in an easy-to-digest form.

Your body is designed to absorb nutrients from whole foods. Natural fruits, vegetables, nuts, seeds, and grains are always the best fuel for the body. As Michael Pollan, author of *Food Rules: An Eater's Manual* (Penguin) says, "If it came from a plant, eat it; if it was made in a plant, don't."

Grape, Orange, and Spinach Motivator

Prep time: 3–4 min • **Blending time:** 2 min • **Yield:** 2 servings

Ingredients	Directions
1 ripe plum 2 kiwis, peeled 2 cups red or green grapes 2 tablespoons ground flaxseed 1 cup fresh orange juice 1 cup water 2 cups baby spinach, loosely packed	*1* Cut the plum and remove the stone, keeping the skin intact. Cut the plum and kiwis into quarters. *2* Combine all the ingredients except the spinach in the blender and secure the lid. *3* Starting at low speed and gradually increasing toward high, blend the ingredients for 45 seconds or until the mixture contains no visible pieces of fruit. *4* Add the spinach and blend again at medium speed for 30 seconds, gradually increasing the speed to high. Blend on high speed for another 15 to 30 seconds or until the entire mixture is smooth. *5* Pour the smoothie into two glasses and enjoy!

Per serving: Calories 283 (From Fat 32); Fat 3.5g (Saturated 0g); Cholesterol 0mg; Sodium 32mg; Carbohydrate 64g (Dietary Fiber 7g); Protein 6g.

Tip: If you don't have time to make fresh-pressed orange juice, use a whole, peeled and seeded orange instead.

Strawberry, Peach, and Maca Prep

Prep time: 3-4 min • **Blending time:** 2 min • **Yield:** 2 servings

Ingredients	Directions
1 ripe peach	*1* Cut the peach and the pear and remove the stone and core, respectively, keeping the skin intact. Cut the flesh into quarters.
1 ripe pear	
1 cup halved strawberries, stems and leaves removed	*2* Combine the peach, pear, strawberries, banana, celery, hemp seed, maca powder, honey, and water in the blender and secure the lid.
1 ripe banana, peeled	
1 stalk celery, roughly chopped	
2 tablespoons hemp seeds	*3* Starting at low speed and gradually increasing toward high, blend the ingredients for 45 seconds or until the mixture contains no visible pieces of fruit.
½ tablespoon maca powder	
1 tablespoon raw honey	
1½ cups water	*4* Remove and discard the stems of the kale leaves. Add the celery greens and kale and blend again at medium speed for 30 seconds, gradually increasing the speed to high. Blend on high speed for another 15 to 30 seconds or until the entire mixture is smooth.
1 cup celery greens, loosely packed	
3 large kale leaves	
	5 Pour the smoothie into two glasses and enjoy!

Per serving: Calories 306 (From Fat 72); Fat 8g (Saturated 0.5g); Cholesterol 0mg; Sodium 77mg; Carbohydrate 56g (Dietary Fiber 11g); Protein 10g.

Tip: You can also add 1 tablespoon of bee pollen in addition to the honey for added protein and immune-boosting nutrients. (Of course, that's only if you aren't allergic to it or to bees or pollen individually, as I discuss earlier in the chapter.)

Tip: Boost the protein in this smoothie even more by adding ½ cup of fresh mung bean, lentil, or alfalfa sprouts in Step 4 with the other greens.

Banana, Spirulina, and Coconut Water Recharge

Prep time: 25 min • **Blending time:** 2 min • **Yield:** 2 servings

Ingredients	*Directions*
2 tablespoons goji berries 2 ripe bananas, peeled 1½ cups pineapple chunks	*1* Place the goji berries in a bowl with ¼ cup of room temperature water. Place in the fridge to soak for at least 20 minutes or overnight.
2 tablespoons ground flaxseed 2 teaspoons spirulina powder ½-inch piece fresh ginger (peeled) 1½ cups coconut water ½ cup water	*2* Combine the goji berries, banana, pineapple, flaxseed, spirulina, ginger, coconut water, and water in the blender and secure the lid.
	3 Starting at low speed and gradually easing toward high, blend the ingredients for 30 to 45 seconds or until smooth.
1 cup mustard greens, loosely packed 1 cup baby spinach, loosely packed	*4* Add the mustard greens and spinach and blend again at medium speed for 30 seconds, gradually increasing the speed to high. Blend on high speed for another 30 seconds or until the entire mixture is smooth.
	5 Pour the smoothie into two glasses and enjoy!

Per serving: Calories 339 (From Fat 36); Fat 4g (Saturated 0.5g); Cholesterol 0mg; Sodium 262mg; Carbohydrate 73g (Dietary Fiber 10g); Protein 8g.

Tip: If you don't have fresh ginger, use ¼ teaspoon of ground ginger instead.

Tip: Mustard greens have a naturally spicy or peppery taste. Taste a leaf before adding it to your smoothie. If you don't like it, use baby spinach or kale instead.

Vary It! Replace the pineapple with fresh mango.

Chia, Raspberry, and Turmeric Zen

Prep time: 25 min • **Blending time:** 2 min • **Yield:** 2 servings

Ingredients	Directions
2 tablespoons chia seeds **½ cup raspberries**	*1* Place the chia seeds in a bowl with ¼ cup of room temperature water. Place in the fridge to soak for at least 20 minutes or overnight.
1 ripe banana, peeled **¼ teaspoon ground turmeric**	*2* Combine all the ingredients except the Swiss chard in the blender and secure the lid.
¼ teaspoon ground cinnamon **1½ cups water**	*3* Starting at low speed and gradually increasing toward high, blend the ingredients for 45 seconds or until the mixture contains no visible pieces of fruit.
4 Swiss chard leaves	*4* Remove and discard the stems of the Swiss chard. Add the Swiss chard and blend again at medium speed for 30 seconds, gradually increasing the speed to high. Blend on high speed for another 15 to 30 seconds or until the entire mixture is smooth.
	5 Pour the smoothie into two glasses and enjoy!

Per serving: Calories 147 (From Fat 45); Fat 5g (Saturated 0.5g); Cholesterol 0mg; Sodium 47mg; Carbohydrate 25g (Dietary Fiber 9g); Protein 4g.

Tip: You can use coconut water instead of water in this recipe for added electrolytes, an especially good idea after an intense hot yoga workout. Add 1 tablespoon of raw honey for a sweeter flavor.

Recovering with anti-inflammatory foods

Muscle soreness after intense exercise usually builds up in the 24 hours after activity. A few different theories attempt to explain this feeling, but the most current one suggests that the exercise causes *microtrauma* to the muscle fibers. In a short period of time, the damaged muscles become swollen and sore. What's the best way to relieve swelling or inflammation? By adding anti-inflammatory foods to your smoothie, of course! Foods such as turmeric, ginger, honey, cinnamon, and fresh fruits and greens are all natural anti-inflammatory foods. Adding these ingredients to your diet before and after exercise helps your muscles repair more quickly and reduces your recovery time between workouts.

High Power Tahini, Date, and Avocado

Prep time: 5–6 min • **Blending time:** 2 min • **Yield:** 2 servings

Ingredients	Directions
½ avocado, peeled and pitted	*1* Combine all the ingredients except the collard greens in the blender and secure the lid.
2 Medjool dates, pitted	
2 ripe bananas, peeled	*2* Starting at low speed and gradually increasing toward high, blend the ingredients for 45 seconds or until smooth.
2 tablespoons hemp seed	
1 tablespoon ground flaxseed	
2 tablespoons sesame tahini	*3* Remove and discard the stems of the collard greens. Add the collard greens and blend again at medium speed for 30 seconds, gradually increasing the speed to high. Blend on high speed for another 15 to 30 seconds or until the entire mixture is smooth.
1 teaspoon maca powder	
1 teaspoon bee pollen (omit if allergic)	
½ teaspoon kelp powder	
1 cup water	
1 cup fresh orange juice	*4* Pour the smoothie into two glasses and enjoy!
4 large collard green leaves	

Per serving: Calories 546 (From Fat 198); Fat 22g (Saturated 2.5g); Cholesterol 0mg; Sodium 15mg; Carbohydrate 79g (Dietary Fiber 13g); Protein 15g.

Tip: Drink this smoothie for strength training recovery and muscle repair.

Tip: If you don't have kelp powder, use spirulina powder instead. You can also use coconut water instead of water in this recipe for added electrolytes.

Staying hydrated

You can eat all the best fruits and vegetables on the planet but still feel tired or have sores muscles if you're dehydrated. Drinking enough water is so important for overall health. In addition to having a smoothie, drink plenty of water throughout the day.

If you're too busy or simply forget to drink water every day, try having two large glasses of water first thing every morning. Even better, add 2 tablespoons of fresh lemon juice or raw apple cider vinegar to each glass and stir well before drinking. The combination will help wake up your stomach and get your digestive enzymes going for the day.

Chapter 15

Green Smoothies for Fertility, Pregnancy, and Beyond

Green smoothies can absolutely help with fertility, pregnancy, and breast-feeding. In my health coaching practice, I had one client who had trouble conceiving for years. In less than six weeks of having a daily green smoothie, she became pregnant naturally! She now has a healthy little boy who happens to love green smoothies, too. In fact, she calls him her "green smoothie baby."

The fruits, greens, and healthy fats in green smoothies provide all sorts of benefits for you and baby at every stage. When you're trying to conceive, that's the time to prepare your body with a nutrient-rich diet and create the most fertile, healthy environment in which your baby can grow. During pregnancy, you're literally eating for two. You need even more nutrients and high-quality fruits and veggies to transfer all that goodness to your baby. And if you choose to breast-feed, the work isn't done! Creating breast milk requires a nutrient-dense diet, too.

This chapter offers green smoothie recipes for fertility, for pregnancy, and for breast-feeding moms. What better time to start eating more fresh fruits and vegetables than when you're bringing a new child into the world? Drinking your fruits and greens in a blended form helps you digest everything more easily. Feel free to share these recipes with your loved ones, too; they're not just for the ladies! Everyone can benefit from added folate, minerals, fiber, chlorophyll, and healthy fats. Here's to good health for your entire family!

The Bee Pollen, Wheatgrass, and Goji Glory smoothie in this chapter calls for bee pollen, which you should leave out if you're allergic to pollen or to bees. Even if you don't have one of these allergies, before including that ingredient in a smoothie check out Chapter 6 for important information on how to determine whether you're sensitive to consuming bee pollen.

Using Smoothies to Boost Fertility

Diet plays an important role in fertility. When you or your partner is ready to conceive, both of you can benefit from drinking green smoothies. Pumpkin seeds and sesame tahini offer high levels of zinc, a natural fertility boost for men and women. For women, leafy greens are a good source of iron and folate. Papaya, blue-berries, oranges, strawberries, and kiwi are high in vitamin C and other antioxidants, and that's important for keeping your immune system strong. And maca powder is known to increase sex drive, so add that to your smoothies to help get things started!

Because you may suffer from morning sickness at the onset of pregnancy, you've actually got more opportunity to get added vita-mins and minerals in your diet before you conceive. Choose your foods wisely and enjoy as much variety as you can now. After you're pregnant, your appetite can change.

The following green smoothie recipes for fertility incorporate a lot of different superfoods, including acai powder, spirulina powder, kelp powder, wheatgrass powder, maca powder, and goji berries. These can all boost your nutrient intake and put your body on the fast track to a healthy pregnancy. Take them during preconception, but after you know you're pregnant, set the superfood powders aside and focus more on whole foods (and the next section of reci-pes for pregnancy). Although no hard evidence indicates that any of the powders are actually dangerous to take during pregnancy, no research has confirmed that they're safe, either. Many women report taking superfoods while pregnant with no adverse effects, but I recommended that you play it safe and avoid them.

Strawberry, Pumpkin Seed, and Royal Jelly

Prep time: 3–4 min • **Blending time:** 2 min • **Yield:** 2 servings

Ingredients	Directions
1½ cups halved strawberries, leaves and stems removed	*1* Combine all the ingredients except the spinach in the blender and secure the lid.
⅓ cup raw pumpkin seeds	
1 ripe banana, peeled	*2* Starting at low speed and gradually increasing toward high, blend the ingredients for 30 to 45 seconds or until the mixture contains no visible pieces of fruit.
1 teaspoon royal jelly	
1½ cups water	
2 cups baby spinach, loosely packed	*3* Add the spinach and blend again at medium speed for 15 to 30 seconds, gradually increasing the speed to high. Blend on high speed for another 15 to 20 seconds or until the entire mixture is smooth.
	4 Pour the smoothie into two glasses and enjoy!

Per serving: Calories 229 (From Fat 108); Fat 12g (Saturated 0g); Cholesterol 0mg; Sodium 31mg; Carbohydrate 27g (Dietary Fiber 6g); Protein 9g.

Note: Royal jelly is a natural secretion from the glands of worker bees, and it's fed to the queen bee for her entire life. This nutrient-dense food helps to strengthen and prepare the queen bee's ovaries to eventually lay millions of eggs in her lifetime. You can easily see why royal jelly is a food known for fertility, and perhaps even one of the most potent natural fertility boosters there is.

Vary It! Try adding 1½ cups of fresh blueberries instead of strawberries. Add ¼ teaspoon of vanilla extract and/or a dash of ground cinnamon for a sweeter taste.

Full-Bodied Almond, Hemp, and Acai

Prep time: 3–4 min • **Blending time:** 2 min • **Yield:** 2 servings

Ingredients	Directions
2 kiwis, peeled	*1* Combine all the ingredients except the Swiss chard in the blender and secure the lid.
1 cup blackberries	
1 tablespoon fresh lime juice	*2* Starting at low speed and gradually increasing toward high, blend the ingredients for 30 to 45 seconds or until the mixture is smooth.
2 tablespoons raw almond butter	
2 tablespoons hemp powder	
1 tablespoon acai powder	*3* Remove and discard the stems of the Swiss chard. Add the Swiss chard and blend again at medium speed for 30 seconds, gradually increasing the speed to high. Blend on high speed for another 15 to 20 seconds or until the entire mixture is smooth.
1½ cups water	
4 Swiss chard leaves	
	4 Pour the smoothie into two glasses and enjoy!

Per serving: Calories 219 (From Fat 99); Fat 11g (Saturated 1g); Cholesterol 0mg; Sodium 48mg; Carbohydrate 26 (Dietary Fiber 10g); Protein 9g.

Vary It! Use 2 cups of red or green grapes instead of kiwis. Add ¼ teaspoon of ground turmeric for an added twist of flavor.

Apple, Tahini, and Maca Abundance

Prep time: 3–4 min • **Blending time:** 2 min • **Yield:** 2 servings

Ingredients	Directions
2 green apples	**1** Cut the apples and remove the cores, keeping the skin intact. Cut the flesh into quarters.
½ avocado, peeled and pitted	
2 tablespoons sesame tahini	**2** Combine the apple, avocado, tahini, dates, spirulina, maca powder, and water in the blender and secure the lid.
2 Medjool dates, pitted	
1 teaspoon spirulina powder	
2 tablespoons maca powder	**3** Starting at low speed and gradually increasing toward high, blend the ingredients for 30 to 45 seconds or until the mixture is smooth.
2½ cups water	
1 cup watercress, loosely packed	
1 cup baby spinach, loosely packed	**4** Add the watercress and spinach and blend again at medium speed for 30 to 45 seconds, gradually increasing the speed to high. Blend on high speed for another 15 to 20 seconds or until the entire mixture is smooth.
	5 Pour the smoothie into two glasses and enjoy!

Per serving: Calories 354 (From Fat 117); Fat 13g (Saturated 2g); Cholesterol 0mg; Sodium 53mg; Carbohydrate 58g (Dietary Fiber 11g); Protein 8g.

Vary It! Try using a banana instead of the avocado for a slightly different taste.

Pomegranate, Kelp, and Orange Infusion

Prep time: 3–4 min • **Blending time:** 2 min • **Yield:** 2 servings

Ingredients	Directions
1 cup pomegranate seeds 1 orange, peeled and seeded	*1* Combine all the ingredients except the kale in the blender and secure the lid.
1 teaspoon kelp powder 2 tablespoons ground flaxseed	*2* Starting at low speed and gradually increasing toward high, blend the ingredients for 30 to 45 seconds or until the mixture is smooth.
1 tablespoon flaxseed oil 1½ cups water 3 large kale leaves	*3* Remove and discard the stems of the kale. Add the kale and blend again at medium speed for 30 seconds, gradually increasing the speed to high. Blend on high speed for another 15 to 20 seconds or until the entire mixture is smooth.
	4 Pour the smoothie into two glasses and enjoy!

Per serving: Calories 255 (From Fat 99); Fat 11g (Saturated 1g); Cholesterol 0mg; Sodium 24mg; Carbohydrate 39g (Dietary Fiber 10g); Protein 6g.

Tip: If you don't have fresh pomegranate seeds, use 2 tablespoons of pomegranate powder instead.

Vary It! Use 1½ cups of coconut water instead of plain water for added electrolytes.

Bee Pollen, Wheatgrass, and Goji Glory

Prep time: 25 min • **Blending time:** 2 min • **Yield:** 2 servings

Ingredients	Directions
2 tablespoons dried goji berries **1 ripe mango** **2 cups pineapple chunks** **1 tablespoon bee pollen (omit if allergic)** **1 teaspoon wheatgrass powder** **2 cups water** **2 large collard green leaves**	*1* Place the goji berries in a bowl with ¼ cup of room temperature water. Place in the fridge to soak for at least 20 minutes or overnight. *2* Peel the mango and cut the flesh away from the stone. *3* Combine all the ingredients except the collard greens in the blender and secure the lid. *4* Starting at low speed and gradually increasing toward high, blend the ingredients for 30 to 45 seconds or until smooth. *5* Remove and discard the stems of the collard greens. Add the greens and blend again at medium speed for 30 to 45 seconds, gradually increasing the speed to high. Blend on high speed for another 15 to 20 seconds or until the entire mixture is smooth. *6* Pour the smoothie into two glasses and enjoy!

Per serving: Calories 313 (From Fat 9); Fat 1g (Saturated 0.5g); Cholesterol 0mg; Sodium 29mg; Carbohydrate 68g (Dietary Fiber 7g); Protein 5g.

Tip: If you don't have mango, use 1 cup of fresh papaya instead.

Meeting Nutrition Needs with Smoothies during Pregnancy

Green smoothies are a healthy choice for mom and baby, so you can consume them regularly throughout your entire pregnancy. Of course, your smoothies should supplement a well-balanced diet full of nutrients, fiber, added protein, and healthy fats.

Green smoothies make a perfect food during pregnancy because their liquid form is easy to digest. The fiber in the fruits and greens helps keep you regular. The fruits are high in vitamins that keep you and your baby strong. Leafy greens are a natural source of folate, and that nutrient is critical for preventing certain birth defects. Greens are also a good source of calcium and magnesium. Consuming healthy fats — especially omega-3 fatty acids, found in flaxseed, chia seeds, and flaxseed oil — is good for your baby's brain health. Selenium (found in walnuts) is also important for your baby's brain development.

Enjoy your smoothie as a snack or with a meal — whatever works best for you — but keep in mind that you should definitely be eating more often while pregnant. Have a green smoothie on-hand when you're shopping, working, visiting friends, or traveling. As soon as you feel hungry, sip your smoothie to keep you hydrated, minimize hunger spells, and stabilize blood sugars.

If you're suffering from morning sickness in the early stages of pregnancy, try drinking small amounts of green smoothie containing ½-inch piece of peeled fresh ginger to calm your stomach. If you're most unwell in the morning hours, drink your green smoothie at night — even before going to bed. Leave a little extra at your bedside and have a few sips every time you get up to use the toilet throughout the night. Waking up hydrated can make an easier to start your day and hopefully reduce any queasiness.

Outstanding Coco-Blueberry and Walnut

Prep time: 3–4 min • **Blending time:** 2 min • **Yield:** 2 servings

Ingredients	Directions
1½ cups blueberries	*1* Combine all the ingredients except the spinach in the blender and secure the lid.
1 ripe banana, peeled	
2 tablespoons coconut oil	*2* Starting at low speed and gradually increasing toward high, blend the ingredients for 30 to 45 seconds or until the mixture is smooth.
6 walnut halves, or 10 walnut pieces (raw, unsalted)	
1½ cups water	
2 cups baby spinach, loosely packed	*3* Add the spinach and blend again at medium speed for 15 to 20 seconds, gradually increasing the speed to high. Blend on high speed for another 15 seconds or until the entire mixture is smooth.
	4 Pour the smoothie into two glasses and enjoy!

Per serving: Calories 343 (From Fat 216); Fat 24g (Saturated 13g); Cholesterol 0mg; Sodium 29mg; Carbohydrate 32g (Dietary Fiber 6g); Protein 2g.

Tip: If you don't have walnuts, use 6 raw, unsalted almonds instead.

Vary It! Instead of blueberries, try 1½ cups of fresh raspberries.

Magnificent Raspberry and Almond Milk

Prep time: 3–4 min • **Blending time:** 2 min • **Yield:** 2 servings

Ingredients	Directions
1 cup raspberries 1 ripe banana, peeled 1 tablespoon blackstrap molasses 1 tablespoon coconut oil 2 cups homemade almond milk ½ cup water 1 cup baby bok choy leaves, loosely packed 1 cup baby spinach, loosely packed	**1** Combine the raspberries, banana, molasses, coconut oil, almond milk, and water in the blender and secure the lid. **2** Starting at low speed and gradually increasing toward high, blend the ingredients for 30 to 45 seconds or until the mixture contains no visible pieces of fruit. **3** Add the bok choy and spinach and blend again at medium speed for 15 to 20 seconds, gradually increasing the speed to high. Blend on high speed for another 15 seconds or until the entire mixture is smooth. **4** Pour the smoothie into two glasses and enjoy!

Per serving: Calories 214 (From Fat 90); Fat 10g (Saturated 6g); Cholesterol 0mg; Sodium 222mg; Carbohydrate 30g (Dietary Fiber 7g); Protein 3g.

Tip: For info on making homemade almond milk, check out Chapter 6.

Vary It! Add 2 tablespoons of unsweetened coconut flakes for a more tropical flavor.

Eat more of these foods when pregnant

Your body needs certain added nutrients during pregnancy. In particular, be sure to increase your intake of the following foods:

✔ Good fats such as almonds, walnuts, and flaxseed oil for added omega-3 fatty acids

✔ Sweet potatoes, carrots, and yellow veggies for beta carotene

✔ Cooked chickpeas, lentils, and black beans for added fiber and protein

✔ Brown rice and other whole grains for B-complex vitamins

✔ Sesame seeds, tahini, and leafy greens for added calcium and zinc

Persimmon and Ginger Happy Morning

Prep time: 25 min • **Blending time:** 2 min • **Yield:** 2 servings

Ingredients	Directions
2 tablespoons chia seeds	**1** Place the chia seeds in a bowl with ¼ cup of room temperature water. Place in the fridge to soak for at least 20 minutes or overnight.
2 ripe persimmons	
1 red delicious or gala apple	
½-inch piece fresh ginger (peeled)	**2** Cut the persimmons; remove the stems and any large seeds, keeping the skin intact. Cut and core the apple, keeping the skin intact; cut the flesh into quarters.
1 tablespoon flaxseed oil	
2 cups water	
1 cup dandelion greens, loosely packed	**3** Combine the chia seeds, persimmon, apple, ginger, flaxseed oil, and water in the blender and secure the lid.
1 cup celery leaves, loosely packed	
	4 Starting at low speed and gradually increasing toward high, blend the ingredients for 30 to 45 seconds or until the mixture contains no visible pieces of fruit.
	5 Add the dandelion greens and celery leaves and blend again at medium speed for 30 seconds, gradually increasing the speed to high. Blend on high speed for another 15 to 30 seconds or until the entire mixture is smooth.
	6 Pour the smoothie into two glasses and enjoy!

Per serving: Calories 257 (From Fat 108); Fat 12g (Saturated 1g); Cholesterol 0mg; Sodium 77mg; Carbohydrate 36g (Dietary Fiber 9g); Protein 5g.

Tip: Although eating the skin of persimmon is okay, some varieties have a rather thick skin and you may find it hard to blend the fruit with the skin on. In that case, peel the skin of the persimmon before adding to the blender in Step 2.

Incredible Apricot, Cherry, and Tahini

Prep time: 3–4 min • **Blending time:** 2 min • **Yield:** 2 servings

Ingredients	Directions
2 ripe apricots 1 cup cherries (pitted) 2 tablespoons sesame tahini 2 tablespoons ground flaxseed 2 cups water 4 baby kale leaves	**1** Cut the apricots and remove the stones, keeping the skin intact. Cut the flesh into quarters. **2** Combine all the ingredients except the kale in the blender and secure the lid. **3** Starting at low speed and gradually increasing toward high, blend the ingredients for 30 to 45 seconds or until the mixture contains no visible pieces of fruit. **4** Add the kale and blend again at medium speed for 15 to 20 seconds, gradually increasing the speed to high. Blend on high speed for another 15 seconds or until the entire mixture is smooth. **5** Pour the smoothie into two glasses and enjoy!

Per serving: Calories 168 (From Fat 99); Fat 11g (Saturated 1g); Cholesterol 0mg; Sodium 29mg; Carbohydrate 16g (Dietary Fiber 5g); Protein 6g.

Tip: You can substitute 4 dried organic apricots (soaked for 20 minutes) or 2 tablespoons of organic dried cherries (soaked for 20 minutes) for the fresh versions of those fruits.

Vary It! Add 1 ripe banana for a creamier texture and taste.

Creamy Avocado, Honey, and Flax

Prep time: 3–4 min • **Blending time:** 2 min • **Yield:** 2 servings

Ingredients	Directions
½ avocado, peeled and pitted	**1** Combine all the ingredients except the Swiss chard in the blender and secure the lid.
2 kiwis, peeled	
2 tablespoons fresh lemon juice	**2** Starting at low speed and gradually increasing toward high, blend the ingredients for 30 to 45 seconds or until the mixture is smooth.
1 tablespoon manuka honey	
2 tablespoons ground flaxseed	
1½ cups water	**3** Remove and discard the stems of the Swiss chard. Add the Swiss chard and blend again at medium speed for 15 to 20 seconds, gradually increasing the speed to high. Blend on high speed for another 15 seconds or until the entire mixture is smooth.
3 Swiss chard leaves	
	4 Pour the smoothie into two glasses and enjoy!

Per serving: Calories 176 (From Fat 72); Fat 8g (Saturated 1g); Cholesterol 0mg; Sodium 49mg; Carbohydrate 28g (Dietary Fiber 6g); Protein 4g.

Vary It! Use 1 fresh peach (stone removed) or 4 to 5 fresh figs instead of the kiwis.

Ingredients to avoid during pregnancy

Though most foods are safe to eat, you should avoid others. Here are some smoothie ingredients to steer clear of when you're eating for two:

- ✔ **Parsley:** At high doses, the oils in parsley can stimulate uterine contractions that can bring on early contractions or induce miscarriage.

- ✔ **Pineapple:** Large amounts of pineapple can affect pregnancy hormones.

- ✔ **Raw sprouts:** Because alfalfa sprouts, sunflower sprouts, and other fresh sprouts can be contaminated with bacteria, avoiding them is your best bet.

- ✔ **Aloe vera, cinnamon, and superfood powders:** Not enough testing has been done to prove the safety or contraindications with these foods; they're just not worth the risk during pregnancy.

Packing Smoothies with Calories and Nutrients while Breast-Feeding

As a nursing mother, you're not finished eating for two just yet! A breast-feeding diet needs to be high in healthy fats and calories to keep your body healthy, strong, and lactating after giving birth. Now is *not* the time to reduce calories or try any extreme weight-loss diets. Restricting calories doesn't allow your body to make nutrient-dense milk, which your baby needs. And actually, your metabolism is working more quickly than ever while breast-feeding just to produce your baby's daily supply of milk. In fact, you get to eat an added 500 calories per day, and you're still likely to lose weight! So let yourself indulge in healthy foods. The green smoothie recipes outlined in this section are all calorie- and nutrient-dense and designed to help you increase your breast-milk production.

Choosing to breast-feed is a very personal choice that depends on many external factors. If you decide to breast-feed, put healthy eating at the top of your agenda. Remember, everything you eat is used to make the milk you feed your baby. Unhealthy eating can make you feel tired and more prone to illness, and it can affect the health of your baby, too. For a healthy breast-feeding diet, choose variety in your fruits, vegetables, nuts, whole grains, and seeds to keep your mineral and vitamin reserves high. Keep in mind that breast-fed babies actually get accustomed to the flavor of foods in their mothers' diets and even develop tastes for those same foods as they grow. So making healthy choices now may help lay the foundation for good eating habits for your child in the future.

Head to www.dummies.com/extras/greensmoothies to find a bonus green smoothie recipe of Amazing Avocado and Pineapple Pizzazz when you're breast-feeding.

Cashew and Blueberry Brilliance

Prep time: 3–4 min • **Blending time:** 2 min • **Yield:** 2 servings

Ingredients	Directions
1 red delicious or gala apple	**1** Cut the apple and remove the core, keeping the skin intact. Cut the flesh into quarters.
1 cup blueberries	
1 ripe banana, peeled	
2 tablespoons raw cashew butter	**2** Combine the apple, blueberries, banana, cashew butter, flaxseed oil, and water in the blender and secure the lid.
1 tablespoon flaxseed oil	
2 cups water	**3** Starting at low speed and gradually increasing toward high, blend the ingredients for 30 to 45 seconds or until the mixture is smooth.
1 cup baby spinach, loosely packed	
1 cup celery leaves, loosely packed	**4** Add the spinach and celery leaves and blend again at medium speed for 15 to 30 seconds, gradually increasing the speed to high. Blend on high speed for another 15 to 20 seconds or until the entire mixture is smooth.
	5 Pour the smoothie into two glasses and enjoy!

Per serving: Calories 307 (From Fat 135); Fat 15g (Saturated 2.5g); Cholesterol 0mg; Sodium 63mg; Carbohydrate 43g (Dietary Fiber 7g); Protein 5g.

Tip: Use 2 tablespoons of coconut oil if you don't have cashew butter.

Vary It! Use ½ avocado (peeled and pitted) instead of the banana.

Peachy Date and Almond Love

Prep time: 3–4 min • **Blending time:** 2 min • **Yield:** 2 servings

Ingredients	Directions
2 ripe peaches	*1* Cut the peaches and remove the stones, keeping the skin intact. Cut the flesh into quarters.
2 Medjool dates, pitted	
2 tablespoons coconut oil	
¼ teaspoon vanilla extract	*2* Combine all the ingredients except the spinach in the blender and secure the lid.
2 tablespoons ground hemp seed	
1½ cups homemade almond milk	*3* Starting at low speed and gradually easing toward high, blend the ingredients for 30 to 45 seconds or until smooth.
2 cups baby spinach, loosely packed	
	4 Add the spinach and blend again at medium speed for 30 to 45 seconds, gradually increasing the speed to high. Blend on high speed for another 15 seconds or until the entire mixture is smooth.
	5 Pour the smoothie into two glasses and enjoy!

Per serving: Calories 364 (From Fat 207); Fat 23g (Saturated 12g); Cholesterol 0mg; Sodium 157mg; Carbohydrate 36g (Dietary Fiber 7g); Protein 8g.

Tip: If you don't have Medjool dates, use 2 tablespoons of manuka honey instead. Chapter 6 has details on making homemade almond milk.

Vary It! Add a banana for a smoother, creamier texture.

Mango-Citrus Afternoon Radiance

Prep time: 3–4 min • **Blending time:** 2 min • **Yield:** 2 servings

Ingredients	Directions
1 ripe mango	**1** Peel the mango and cut the flesh away from the stone.
1 orange, peeled and seeded	
1 cup halved strawberries, stems and leaves removed	**2** Combine all the ingredients except the collard greens in the blender and secure the lid.
2 tablespoons ground flaxseed	
1 tablespoon flaxseed oil	**3** Starting at low speed and gradually increasing toward high, blend the ingredients for 30 to 45 seconds or until the mixture is smooth.
1 tablespoon coconut oil	
2 cups water	
2 large collard green leaves	**4** Remove and discard the stems of the collard greens. Add the greens and blend again at medium speed for 30 seconds, gradually increasing the speed to high. Blend on high speed for another 30 seconds or until the entire mixture is smooth.
	5 Pour the smoothie into two glasses and enjoy!

Per serving: Calories 325 (From Fat 153); Fat 17g (Saturated 7g); Cholesterol 0mg; Sodium 9mg; Carbohydrate 41g (Dietary Fiber 9g); Protein 5g.

Vary It! Instead of strawberries, try a ripe banana (peeled).

Sunflower, Banana, and Cinnamon Sunrise

Prep time: 25 min • **Blending time:** 2 min • **Yield:** 2 servings

Ingredients	Directions
2 tablespoons chia seeds	*1* Place the chia seeds in a bowl with ¼ cup of room temperature water. Place in the fridge to soak for at least 20 minutes or overnight.
⅓ cup raw sunflower seeds	
1 ripe banana, peeled	
2 tablespoons sesame tahini	*2* Combine all the ingredients except the romaine in the blender and secure the lid.
½ teaspoon ground cinnamon	
1½ cups water	*3* Starting at low speed and gradually increasing toward high, blend the ingredients for 30 to 45 seconds or until smooth.
5 large romaine lettuce leaves	
	4 Remove and discard the stalks of the romaine. Add the romaine and blend again at medium speed for 15 to 30 seconds, gradually increasing the speed to high. Blend on high speed for another 30 seconds or until the entire mixture is smooth.
	5 Pour the smoothie into two glasses and enjoy!

Per serving: Calories 356 (From Fat 225); Fat 25g (Saturated 3g); Cholesterol 0mg; Sodium 16mg; Carbohydrate 29g (Dietary Fiber 11g); Protein 10g.

Vary It! Add 1 apple or 1 pear in addition to the banana for some extra fiber and flavor. Instead of cinnamon, try a small piece of fresh ginger (½ inch or less, peeled).

Chapter 16

Green Smoothies for Detoxification

In This Chapter

▶ Understanding how detox works

▶ Getting the lowdown on one- and three-day green smoothie cleanses

▶ Whipping up smoothies for your cleanse

*T*hink about how much time you spend taking showers, brushing your teeth, and grooming your hair and nails, all for the purpose of removing dirt, feeling clean, smelling fresh, and looking good. But how much time do you spend cleaning the *inside* of your body? The modern world is a pretty toxic place. Every day, you breathe chemicals in the air, put chemicals on your skin, and eat chemicals in your food. Packaged foods alone contain more than 3,000 food additives, and that doesn't even include all the different pesticides sprayed on fruits and vegetables. Even if you eat relatively well, you can still overload your body with internal toxins.

In this chapter, I highlight key symptoms to help you know whether you need to do a detox, show you how to do one, and let you in on what to expect. And if you decide to give it a try, I outline guidelines and recipes for doing a one-day or three-day cleanse at home. Whatever detox program you choose, make sure it feels right for you. Don't force yourself to do anything if it doesn't feel right.

 If you suffer from preexisting medical conditions, consult your doctor before starting any type of detox program. The cleanses in this chapter aren't recommended for pregnant or breast-feeding mothers or for children under age 18. Refer to Chapter 15 for information on green smoothies for fertility, pregnancy, and breast-feeding. Chapter 11 lists green smoothie recipes for kids.

Cleaning Your Body from the Inside Out

To keep a car running well, you don't just wash the outside periodically; you take it in for regular maintenance checks. You get an oil change, maybe replace a tire or two, and make sure the engine is clean and working okay. Otherwise, the old oil quickly gets thick and dirty, putting stress on the whole engine. Over time, an unserviced car is more likely to break down, have engine problems, and require more hours at the shop getting fixed.

It's a simple analogy: Your body is the car. Doing a detox is your maintenance check to help you avoid costly visits to the doctor. If you clean your body from the inside out by doing some type of regular detox program, you're getting a mini tune-up and practicing preventative maintenance for your health.

Catching common signs you need to detox

If you suffer from three or more of the following conditions, you're a very good candidate for doing a cleanse:

- Constipation, excessive gas, and/or bloating
- Indigestion and/or acid reflux
- Body odor, bad breath, and/or bad-smelling stools
- Insomnia, light sleep, or sleep that isn't restful
- Headaches or migraines
- Joint aches and pains
- Low energy/fatigue throughout the day
- Poor skin, acne, or rashes
- Thinning hair or brittle nails
- Decreased sex drive
- Excess weight and/or trouble losing weight
- Dark circles under your eyes or puffy eyes
- Frequent colds, flus, or mucous congestion
- Allergies or hay fever

Consult with your doctor and continue to take any prescription medication during the detox program.

What's the difference? Detoxing, cleansing, and fasting

The terms *detox, fast,* and *cleanse* get thrown around a lot these days, often in ways that don't quite match their original meanings. For example, the word *detox* used to apply specifically to ridding the body of drug or alcohol addiction, but now it describes purifying the body from any type of toxic buildup. You may even notice advertising for emotional detox or relationship detox, referring to programs designed to clear old emotional baggage.

Usually, the terms *detox* and *cleanse* are used interchangeably. You can do a raw food cleanse, a liver detox, a skin detox, or a colon cleanse, among many others. Some programs use additional herbal supplements and special fiber drinks or recommend self-administered enemas or colonics, depending on the type of cleanse. To find out more about the process of detox, read *Detox For Dummies* by Caroline Shreeve (John Wiley and Sons, Inc.).

The term *fasting,* in its purest sense, means abstaining from all food in any form and drinking only water for a period of time. But that term is used more loosely these days. You may see people talking about a *juice fast* or a *smoothie fast* where they drink only fresh juices or smoothies for the duration of the fast. *Warning:* The original water-only fast (now called *water fasting*) can be dangerous and isn't recommended without the guidance of a health care provider.

Recognizing why getting rid of excess toxins is important

Your body goes through a natural process of detox on a daily basis. The lungs bring oxygen in with each inhale and release carbon dioxide with each exhale. The liver filters toxins in the blood, the kidneys and skin release acid buildup, and the colon gets rid of solid waste. If the body can eliminate all of that on its own, what's the point of butting in? Why not just let Mother Nature do her job?

The main problem in letting nature take its course is that you're simply putting more in than is going out. The average diet today is heavily loaded with chemical additives, flavorings, coloring agents, pesticides, herbicides, fungicides, and other toxic chemicals that overburden the body. During cleansing and similar programs, the *organs of elimination* — the colon, liver, kidneys, lungs, and skin — are able to eliminate large amounts of these accumulated metabolic wastes and poisons.

The purpose of doing a detox or cleanse is to give all your organs a chance to catch up on internal housekeeping. Have you ever tried to clean your house while people were walking through it? Their feet track dirt all over the floor, their hands touch everything, and you can't even clean the old mess before new mess forms. And even if you clean your house regularly, dust and dirt still gather under and behind furniture. Giving your body just a short break from that constant exposure allows your organs to clear out the buildup without adding more on top of it and provides the health equivalent of a good spring cleaning. Moving forward, all your organs work better, which means your energy levels, immune system, metabolism, and digestive system all improve, too.

Green Smoothie Detox: One Day per Week

If you want to try a detox but are too busy or just aren't ready to make the three-day plunge outlined later in this chapter, doing a green smoothie cleanse one day a week is the perfect option for you.

Here's how it works: Pick a day that works best for you and make that your *detox day.* I like to do my weekly cleanse on Monday. That lets me have some fun on the weekend but stops me from letting any weekend indulgences run over into the week. I like to think of it as a mini reset button to get my body cleaned out and my mind prepared for a productive and healthy week ahead.

For the entire day, drink plenty of water and only green smoothies, choosing detox recipes from this chapter. Try to have one smoothie serving every two to three hours throughout the day. Avoid all coffee, alcohol, and solid food. You should quickly feel energized and see less puffiness (inflammation) in your body and face after just a few hours. You may sleep better that night and wake up the next day feeling more refreshed and experiencing easy-to-pass stools.

I don't recommend trying a one-day detox if you're under extreme stress or have an exceptionally busy day. Skipping a week or even a month until your schedule clears again is okay.

Even if you can manage only one one-day detox per month, that's still better than not doing any cleanse at all! To help you remember when to do your monthly cleanse, choose a routine such as the first day of the month, every first Monday, or every full moon. Do what you can. You can always add more days later.

Note: If you're wondering whether you can add green juice to the program as well, the answer is "of course you can!" But you don't have to, and you don't need to. The green smoothie detox is designed for green smoothies. Its purpose is to add lots of fiber to your body to really give your colon a good cleanse. Green smoothies are full of fiber, but a green juice has no fiber. And who wants to clean a juicer *and* a blender anyway? For this detox, I recommend you keep it simple and drink only green smoothies. (Chapter 1 has the details on the difference between a smoothie and juice.)

Green Smoothie Detox: Simple Three-Day Cleanse

This three-day program is designed to be gentle, and you can do it while working. That said, slowing down during a detox and allowing your body time to rest is still a good idea. Starting on the weekend is a great strategy; that way, you get two days of rest and have only the last day of the cleanse to work or go to school.

Take some time to try other recipes in this book, learn how to use your blender, and get comfortable with making smoothies before starting this three-day cleanse. After you start the cleanse, you don't need any added stress.

Making your detox shopping list

Each recipe in this chapter has a different detox effect on the body, so for a first-timer, it's best that you try all the recipes and not just pick the ones you like. The next time you do the cleanse, you can adjust your plan according to your taste. With that in mind, here's what you need for your three-day cleanse (try to buy organic if possible):

- 3 red apples
- 3 pears
- 1 pineapple
- 1 papaya
- 1 watermelon
- 2 cucumbers
- 3 kiwis
- 4 limes
- 4 lemons
- 6 oranges
- 12 bananas
- 2 pints of blueberries
- 1 bunch of fresh mint
- 1 bunch of fresh parsley
- 1 bunch of fresh cilantro
- 1 bunch of collard greens
- 1 bunch of kale
- 1 bunch of dandelion greens
- 1 bunch of spinach
- 1 bunch of celery leaves (or stalks with leaves)
- 2 bunches of watercress
- 6 Medjool dates
- 12 tablespoons of ground flaxseed

- 6 tablespoons of chia seeds

- 3 tablespoons of spirulina powder

- 3 teaspoons of chlorella powder

- 3 tablespoons of extra-virgin olive oil

- 2 bottles of 100-percent coconut water

- 6 tablespoons of 100-percent aloe vera juice

- 1½ teaspoons of ground turmeric

- 1 teaspoon cayenne pepper

- 1 large piece of fresh ginger

Walking through the detox, day by day

The three-day green smoothie detox program works like this:

- Drink only green smoothies and water. Herbal tea with no added milk or sugar is also okay. Avoid coffee, alcohol, soft drinks, or sugary drinks.

- Have a green smoothie every two to three hours.

- Make each day's smoothies in advance or throughout the day — whatever works best for you. If you make your smoothies ahead of time, remember to store them in the fridge.

- Avoid solid foods.

- Try not to smoke.

- Continue to take all prescription medications.

To maximize your results, have a plan for before, during, and after you detox, and keep the following in mind:

1. **Two days before the detox:** Eliminate coffee, soft drinks, salty foods, and refined sugar as best you can. This step helps reduce your cleansing reactions and prepares your body gently for the detox.

2. **One day before the detox:** Buy all the ingredients you need and have everything at home, on-hand, and ready to go. Cancel any unnecessary appointments and try to make time for yourself.

3. **During the detox:** Spend time outdoors in the sun or in nature, read a book, or watch some health DVDs. Basically, slow down and enjoy the process. Take a hot bath with 1 to 2 cups of Epsom salts (magnesium sulfate) to help

your muscles relax. Drink plenty of water. Try not to watch any violent movies or TV shows. Avoid negative conversations. Fill your mind with positive, happy thoughts.

4. **After the detox:** Eat light foods on the day you break your fast. Have a bowl of fresh seasonal fruit in the morning. At lunch, eat a salad or steamed vegetables. If you're feeling well by dinner, you can have some cooked grains (such as brown rice or red quinoa) and steamed vegetables. Keep drinking plenty of water. By the second day of eating, you can resume your normal diet, which is hopefully a bit healthier after your detox than it was before!

Sticking with it for three days

The hardest part of doing a three-day cleanse is staying committed to it. If you decide to do this detox, stand strong against cravings. The other foods will be there your whole life, and your life will be even longer to enjoy them if you stay fit and healthy!

If you manage to do three days, congratulate yourself for a job well done. You've given yourself a wonderful gift: the gift of good health.

Managing your reactions

As your body starts to stir up and release toxins during a detox, you'll likely feel some mild reactions. The most common symptoms are

- ✔ Headache
- ✔ Mild nausea
- ✔ Fatigue

Usually the feelings pass rather quickly, especially if you drink plenty of water. Practicing deep breathing helps. Fresh ginger tea is good for nausea. Placing a dab of peppermint oil under your nose and at each temple helps reduce the severity of a headache. Taking an Epsom salt bath is good for muscle tension. Give your body time to rest. If you have any serious concerns, be sure to seek medical attention.

Some people experience lightheadedness during a detox. Be sure to stand up *slowly* every time you get up.

Be gentle with yourself, and don't force yourself to continue if you start to really feel unwell. If you stop after one or two days, be proud of what you completed. Remember, one or two days of detox is better than no detox at all! You can always try for the full three days next time.

Common questions about the three-day green smoothie detox

Here are the answers to some frequently asked questions about the three-day smoothie detox:

✔ **How often should I do this cleanse?**

Ideally, you should do this detox program every six months (twice a year), but I recommend once a year at minimum. I like to do one detox in January as a kick-off to a healthy year and another one toward the end of summer to feel healthy and strong for the winter. Some people like to do one detox at the spring solstice and one at the fall solstice. I even know people who like to detox on their birthday as a gift to themselves for good health!

✔ **Can I exercise during the detox?**

You get better results with the detox if you let your body use any extra energy on the inside, working to clean your blood, lymphatic system, and elimination organs. Exercise externalizes your energy and doesn't leave much left for cleansing. Don't force yourself to work out just because that's what you normally do. If you feel energetic, you can practice gentle yoga and stretching or do light cardio such as walking or jogging. If you become lightheaded, though, stop immediately. I don't recommend any extreme cardio (such as spinning), excessive sweating (such as from hot yoga), or strength training with weights. If the idea of skipping workouts concerns you, remember: It's only for three days.

✔ **Do I need to get a colonic/enema during the detox?**

No. Because green smoothies have plenty of fiber, you should be going to the toilet naturally (and probably more than usual) during the cleanse. That's a good sign that your colon is getting a good cleanse. There's no need to do a colonic or enema as well.

✔ **What if I feel hungry?**

If you feel hungry during the cleanse, drink more green smoothies. Have two servings at one time. Drink a smoothie every one and a half to two hours rather than every two to three hours. Drink more water, too. Sometimes hunger is a sign of dehydration.

✔ **Can I go longer than three days?**

Yes! If you're feeling good and you want to continue, you can do this program for up to seven to ten days.

No more S.A.D. eating!

S.A.D. is an acronym for the *Standard American Diet,* which is a diet low in fiber and plant-based foods but high in refined sugar, refined carbohydrates, processed foods, fried food, saturated fats, and cholesterol. Problems with this diet include the following:

✔ It's one of the major factors contributing to *metabolic syndrome,* a condition characterized by increased risk of insulin resistance, high blood pressure, and cholesterol imbalance.

✔ It's the main reason Americans are plagued by higher rates of obesity, heart disease, high cholesterol, and Type 2 diabetes.

✔ It's responsible for increasing the risk of certain cancers and intestinal disorders.

What's even sadder is that other countries around the world have adopted the S.A.D. style of eating and are now experiencing the same increased rates of obesity, heart disease, and Type 2 diabetes as the United States.

To protect yourself from increased risk of metabolic syndrome, you have to make a long-term shift away from S.A.D. foods and toward more dietary fiber and plant-based foods. Use one of the green smoothie cleanses in this chapter as a mini reboot to jump-start this change. From there, drink one green smoothie a day; as your body finally gets the minerals, fiber, and chlorophyll it needs, you'll see how you start to crowd out the S.A.D. foods naturally.

Morning Liver Flush

Prep time: 5 min • **Blending time:** 2 min • **Yield:** 2 servings

Ingredients	Directions
2 oranges, peeled and seeded	*1* Combine the oranges, banana, lemon juice, olive oil, ginger, turmeric, cayenne, and water in the blender and secure the lid.
1 ripe banana, peeled	
¼ cup fresh lemon juice	
1 tablespoon extra-virgin olive oil	*2* Starting at low speed and gradually increasing toward high, blend the ingredients for 30 to 45 seconds or until the mixture is smooth.
½-inch piece fresh ginger (peeled)	
¼ teaspoon ground turmeric	*3* Add the dandelion greens and spinach and blend again at medium speed for 30 seconds, gradually increasing the speed to high. Blend on high speed for another 15 to 30 seconds or until the entire mixture is smooth.
Dash cayenne pepper	
1½ cups water	
1 cup dandelion greens, loosely packed	*4* Pour the smoothie into two glasses and enjoy!
1 cup spinach, loosely packed	

Per serving: Calories 223 (From Fat 72); Fat 8g (Saturated 1g); Cholesterol 0mg; Sodium 44mg; Carbohydrate 33g (Dietary Fiber 6g); Protein 4g.

Tip: If you don't have fresh ginger, use ¼ teaspoon of ground ginger instead. If you have fresh turmeric, you can use ¼ teaspoon of it instead of ground turmeric. Look for fresh dandelion greens at your local farmers' market or health food supermarket.

Tip: If you're feeling good on day three of a three-day cleanse, you can try this smoothie without the banana for a stronger liver cleanse.

Happy Belly Enzymes

Prep time: 5 min • **Blending time:** 2 min • **Yield:** 2 servings

Ingredients	Directions
1½ cups chopped papaya, seeded and peeled (reserve 5 seeds)	*1* Crush the papaya seeds. Place them on a cutting board and press them with the broad side of a knife blade until they break down.
1 cup pineapple chunks	
1 ripe banana, peeled	*2* Combine the papaya seeds and all the ingredients except the kale in the blender and secure the lid.
1 tablespoon fresh lime juice	
2 tablespoons ground flaxseed	
1 tablespoon aloe vera juice	*3* Starting at low speed and gradually increasing toward high, blend the ingredients for 30 to 45 seconds or until the mixture is smooth.
1½ cups water	
3 large kale leaves	
	4 Remove and discard the kale stems. Add the kale and blend again at medium speed for 30 seconds, gradually increasing the speed to high. Blend on high speed for another 15 to 30 seconds or until the entire mixture is smooth.
	5 Pour the smoothie into two glasses and enjoy!

Per serving: Calories 220 (From Fat 27); Fat 3g (Saturated 0g); Cholesterol 0mg; Sodium 37mg; Carbohydrate 48g (Dietary Fiber 7g); Protein 4g.

Tip: A single papaya has lots and lots of seeds. Set aside a few tablespoons of the papaya seeds leftover when you cut up the papaya in this recipe and keep them handy for the rest of your cleanse. You can store them in the refrigerator in a small glass jar or container.

Body Balance

Prep time: 25 min • **Blending time:** 2 min • **Yield:** 2 servings

Ingredients	Directions
2 tablespoons chia seeds 1 red delicious or gala apple 1 ripe pear 2 Medjool dates, pitted 2 tablespoons ground flaxseed ½-inch piece fresh ginger (peeled) 1 teaspoon spirulina powder 1 tablespoon fresh lemon juice 1 cup coconut water ½ cup water 1 cup parsley, loosely packed 1 cup celery leaves, loosely packed	*1* Place the chia seeds in a bowl with ¼ cup of room temperature water. Place in the fridge to soak for at least 20 minutes or overnight. *2* Cut the apple and pear and remove the cores, keeping the skin intact. Cut the flesh into quarters. *3* Combine the chia seeds, apple, pear, dates, flaxseed, ginger, spirulina, lemon juice, coconut water, and water in the blender and secure the lid. *4* Starting at low speed and gradually increasing toward high, blend the ingredients for 30 to 45 seconds or until the mixture contains no visible pieces of fruit. *5* Add the parsley and celery leaves and blend again at medium speed for 30 seconds, gradually increasing the speed to high. Blend on high speed for another 30 seconds or until the entire mixture is smooth. *6* Pour the smoothie into two glasses and enjoy!

Per serving: Calories 335 (From Fat 72); Fat 8g (Saturated 1g); Cholesterol 0mg; Sodium 212mg; Carbohydrate 65g (Dietary Fiber 17g); Protein 9g.

Tip: If you don't have fresh ginger, use ¼ teaspoon of ground ginger instead. If you don't have coconut water, use 1½ cups of water plus 1 tablespoon of coconut oil.

Vary It! Instead of ginger, you can use ¼ teaspoon of ground cinnamon. Instead of pear, use a ripe banana or 1½ cups of red or green grapes.

Heavy Metal Detox

Prep time: 5 min • **Blending time:** 2 min • **Yield:** 2 servings

Ingredients	*Directions*
1½ cups pineapple chunks 1 kiwi, peeled 1 ripe banana, peeled 1 tablespoon fresh lime juice ¼ teaspoon ground turmeric 1 teaspoon chlorella powder 1½ cups water 3 large collard green leaves 1 cup cilantro, loosely packed	*1* Combine the pineapple, kiwi, banana, lime juice, turmeric, chlorella, and water in the blender and secure the lid. *2* Starting at low speed and gradually increasing toward high, blend the ingredients for 30 to 45 seconds or until the mixture contains no visible pieces of fruit. *3* Remove and discard the collard green stems. Add the cilantro and collard greens and blend again at medium speed for 30 seconds, gradually increasing the speed to high. Blend on high speed for another 15 to 30 seconds or until the entire mixture is smooth. *4* Pour the smoothie into two glasses and enjoy!

Per serving: Calories 248 (From Fat 4); Fat 0.5g (Saturated 0g); Cholesterol 0mg; Sodium 26mg; Carbohydrate 56g (Dietary Fiber 6g); Protein 4g.

Tip: If you don't have chlorella powder, use spirulina powder instead.

Vary It! Instead of kiwi, try 1 cup of chopped mango.

Kidney and Skin Cleanse

Prep time: 5 min • **Blending time:** 2 min • **Yield:** 2 servings

Ingredients	Directions
2 cups chopped watermelon	*1* Combine the watermelon, blueberries, cucumber, banana, lime juice, aloe vera, and water in the blender and secure the lid.
1 cup blueberries	
½ cucumber, peeled	
1 ripe banana, peeled	*2* Starting at low speed and gradually increasing toward high, blend the ingredients for 30 to 45 seconds or until the mixture contains no visible pieces of fruit.
¼ cup fresh lime juice	
1 tablespoon aloe vera juice	
1 cup water	*3* Add the mint and watercress and blend again at medium speed for 30 seconds, gradually increasing the speed to high. Blend on high speed for another 15 to 30 seconds or until the entire mixture is smooth.
3 mint leaves	
2 cups watercress, loosely packed	
	4 Pour the smoothie into two glasses and enjoy!

Per serving: Calories 164 (From Fat 9); Fat 1g (Saturated 0g); Cholesterol 0mg; Sodium 23mg; Carbohydrate 41g (Dietary Fiber 5g); Protein 3g.

Tip: Refer to Chapter 6 for information on what types of aloe vera are safe to ingest.

Part V
The Part of Tens

the
part of
tens

In this part . . .

✔ Get up to speed with the most common myths surrounding green smoothies and cut straight through to the facts.

✔ Lay to rest the idea that only expensive blenders make green smoothies and gain new confidence in the smoothie making power of your household blender.

✔ Discover ways to increase the protein, calcium, or iron in your smoothies.

✔ Get answers to the most frequently asked questions about green smoothies, including how to handle gas and bloating and whether it's possible to overdo it with smoothies.

Chapter 17

Ten Green Smoothie Myths Debunked

. . . .

In This Chapter

▶ Busting misconceptions about the dangers of green smoothie ingredients

▶ Setting the record straight on making and drinking smoothies

. . . .

*I*f you have any doubts about how green smoothies can benefit your health, this chapter is for you. I present the ten most popular myths about green smoothies to help you separate fact from fiction. After you read through these pages, you'll be better prepared to answer questions from your family, friends, and coworkers, too.

Green Smoothies Are Too High in Calories

Absolutely untrue! With so many combinations of ingredients, you can alter any green smoothie recipe to match your caloric needs.

To make your green smoothie lower in calories, try the following:

✔ Avoid high-fat ingredients such as avocado, coconut oil, almond milk, cashew butter, tahini, and Brazil nuts.

✔ Minimize dried fruits, which are naturally high in sugar.

✔ Increase low-calorie ingredients, such as cucumber, tomato, red bell pepper, lemons, berries, celery greens, leafy greens, raw apple cider vinegar, and cinnamon.

✔ Add more water to your recipe to dilute the smoothie, giving you more volume to drink with fewer calories per serving.

Green smoothies are full of fiber, and research has shown that a high-fiber diet is good for weight loss because the fiber makes you feel fuller longer and helps control cravings by balancing blood sugar levels. But you can't expect to eat a high-calorie smoothie

packed with high-fat ingredients and lose weight. By choosing the right ingredients for your health goals, you'll fast-track your results.

Green Smoothies Are Too High in Iron

Green leafy vegetables are good plant-based sources of iron that don't raise your cholesterol levels or increase your risk of cardio-vascular disease. But people often worry that greens are too high in iron. Unless you have a medical or genetic condition that causes your body to retain iron, overdosing on iron from green smoothies is extremely unlikely. Actually, the iron from plant-based sources isn't readily *bioavailable* (meaning your body can't access it), and that's exactly why most vegans and vegetarians need to supplement their diets with additional iron.

Still worried about those greens? Consider the following: According to the FDA, the recommended daily allowance of iron for adults is between 8 and 15 milligrams; the Institute of National Health pegs the maximum daily upper limit of iron as 45 milligrams for adults. Now look at the iron content of a smoothie with ingredients that are all naturally high in iron:

- 1 tablespoon spirulina powder: 2 milligrams
- 2 cups raw kale: 2 milligrams
- 2 cups raw spinach: 1.62 milligrams
- 2 fresh apricots: 0.28 milligrams
- 1 cup fresh cherries (pitted): 0.55 milligrams
- 2 tablespoons molasses: 2 milligrams

A green smoothie with all these plant-based sources of iron has a total of only 9.45 milligrams of iron, nowhere near the maximum daily limit. A green smoothie is actually the perfect way to get the right amount of iron you need for the day.

Green Smoothies Have Too Much Oxalic Acid

Some people suggest that the oxalic acid in leafy green veggies can increase your risk of kidney stones. In fact, studies show that the real risk factors for kidney stones are not drinking enough water, suffering from magnesium deficiency, and not having enough calcium in your diet.

True, certain leafy greens, such as spinach, Swiss chard, beet greens, kale, and collard greens, are high in oxalic acid. If you suffer from kidney disease or have only one kidney, minimize your intake of these greens. Leafy greens that are low in oxalic acid include lettuce greens, bok choy, celery, and all fresh herbs except parsley.

A healthy individual should have no problem with the oxalic acid in certain greens. Keep in mind that green smoothies are a mixture of fresh fruits and greens, and the combination of these two types of foods helps to *alkalize* (neutralize) the effects of oxalic acid. You're much more likely to get into trouble with oxalate foods if you eat them on their own without any alkaline foods to balance the acid.

Green Leafy Vegetables Are Toxic

Leafy green vegetables contain very small amounts of *phytotoxins* as a natural defense mechanism to protect the plant from predators. Without them, a plant would taste so appealing that animals would eat all its leaves, and the plant would die.

However, you'd have to eat large entire bunches of kale or spinach every single day for months at a time to feel some type of toxic effect. In the green smoothie recipes in this book, you're eating a maximum of 2 cups of leafy greens, and that's certainly nowhere near an amount to be considered toxic. Remember that moderation and variety are the keys to success with any healthy diet.

You Can Overdose on Vitamins A and K in Smoothies

Your body makes vitamin A as needed from the beta carotene found in orange fruits and dark leafy green vegetables. If your body has enough vitamin A, it won't make any more, so you run no risk of overdosing on vitamin A from plant-based foods. If you eat too much beta carotene (which most commonly happens from juicing high beta carotene foods such as carrots), your skin will simply develop an orange or yellow hue from the excess beta carotene stored in the fat cells of your skin. This effect is harmless (though maybe not so physically attractive).

Overdosing on beta carotene in a green smoothie is virtually impossible because in a smoothie, you still have all the fiber intact. The fiber in a smoothie keeps all vitamin concentrations at lower levels than in a juice with no fiber.

As for vitamin K, most people are actually deficient, leaving them at higher risk for tooth decay, osteoporosis, cardiovascular disease, dementia, and certain types of cancer. Getting more vitamin K from leafy greens in a green smoothie can actually help prevent these diseases. Just know that not all vitamin K is created equal. The natural forms of vitamin K are K1 and K2, and only vitamin K1 is present in plants (especially in green vegetables). K3 is a synthetic form of vitamin K and can be dangerous in high doses, which is why most health practitioners don't recommend vitamin K supplements. There's no known toxicity risk with consuming large amounts of vitamin K1 in natural, whole foods.

Chewing Your Food Is Better for Digestion

The real issue here isn't chewing versus drinking your food; it's chewing completely versus not chewing completely. Chewing your food is very important for good digestion because during chewing, your saliva releases enzymes that help digest and break down your food. But people today eat too fast — on the go, while talking, while driving, or on the phone — and the result is that they're swallowing huge mouthfuls of food at a time. The stomach is forced to release more and more acids in an effort to break down the food. What follows is indigestion, low absorption, poor elimination, or any combination of the three.

In an ideal world, you should drink your foods and chew your juices. When you eat, chew so many times that your food becomes liquid, and then swallow. When you drink, keep the liquid in your mouth, swishing back and forth slowly to release the enzymes in your saliva before swallowing. Green smoothies are the perfect solution, because the blender can do the chewing for you, especially for fibrous leafy greens.

Green Smoothies Require an Expensive Blender

As long as you treat your blender right, you can make a green smoothie in any household blender. The trick to using a normal blender is this: Add fruits and water first. Blend. Then add your leafy greens and blend again. That's it! As long as you have a good liquid base before you add your greens, your inexpensive blender will work. I've been teaching green smoothie classes for years with a $35 blender on purpose to show my students that it can be done!

Turn to Chapter 2 for a complete breakdown of all the features to look for in a blender and how to choose the best blender for green smoothies.

The Blender's Heat Destroys the Enzymes in a Green Smoothie

Enzymes are destroyed when a food is heated to a temperature of 118 degrees Fahrenheit or above. For reference, an average bathtub is heated to about 100 to 105 degrees, and anything over 120 degrees is considered too hot to touch. If your blender is heating the smoothie enough to kill the enzymes, your smoothie should feel too hot to drink and almost too hot to touch after blending. In all my years of making smoothies and using different types of blenders from all over the world, I've never made a smoothie that felt too hot to drink and certainly never one that was too hot to touch.

Practice good blending skills by blending water and fruits first before blending greens, as I explain in the preceding section. Always start blending at a low speed and gradually increase to high speed. Minimize your blending time to 2 minutes for smoothies. These steps help reduce the temperature of your blender motor and keep the enzymes in your green smoothie intact!

A Store-Bought Green Smoothie Is Just as Good as a Homemade One

Hopefully, this book has sold you on the idea of drinking more green smoothies, but perhaps you're so not keen on making them at home. Maybe you've noticed some healthy-looking bottled green drinks at your local convenience store, and you're thinking about going the store-bought route for your daily dose of greens. Hold that thought.

Take a moment to check the ingredients label on that store-bought smoothie, and you'll understand why making your green smoothie at home is always well worth the effort. The main ingredients in a store-bought smoothie are usually apple juice and pineapple juice. What does that mean? The manufacturers bought cheap, artificially flavored apple and pineapple juices to use as the base of your so-called health drink. They didn't use whole apples and pineapples like you would at home. Artificial juices can contain added sugar, and because the sugar is already in the juice, the label can still say *no added sugar*. That's some sneaky food label trickery!

Keep reading the ingredients, and you'll probably also see the term *natural flavors*. Technically, food companies can put just about anything they want under that term because the word *natural* isn't regulated on food labels at all. And although superfoods like wheatgrass and spirulina may be included, if they're not labeled *organic,* they may well contain extras such as heavy metals or added fillers.

Don't be fooled by nice labels and good advertising. Taking a few minutes to make your smoothie at home is a guarantee that you know exactly what's in your smoothie and your ingredients are of the highest quality. You're worth it!

Some People Shouldn't Drink Green Smoothies

The only reason you shouldn't drink green smoothies is if you shouldn't be eating food. Yes, really! There are endless combinations of fruits and greens to match everyone's individual needs. If you have health conditions with diet restrictions, you can adjust your ingredients accordingly. If you suffer from food allergies, use alternative ingredients wherever necessary. For green smoothie recipes for specific ailments, refer to Chapters 12 and 13.

Chapter 18

Ten Common Questions about Green Smoothies

In This Chapter

▶ Fine-tuning smoothie ingredients to meet your weight and nutritional goals

▶ Considering green juices and multivitamins

*I*f you're new to the green smoothie game, you probably have a lot of questions. In this chapter, I answer the ten most frequently asked questions about green smoothies. Think of this chapter as a crash course in green smoothies and a reminder of all the health benefits you can experience when you start adding this outstanding health drink to your daily routine.

How Can I Lose Weight on Green Smoothies?

It's easy! Drink your green smoothie as a replacement meal for one or two meals each day. For example, choose a green smoothie from Chapter 8 for breakfast, enjoy a green smoothie from Chapter 9 for lunch, and eat a normal healthy meal for dinner. You can follow this regimen for four to six weeks or however long you need to reach your weight loss goal. Avoid adding too much fat to your smoothies to keep the calorie count low. Minimize your use of coconut oil, avocado, nuts, nut milks, almond butter, and tahini.

Because green smoothies are so high in fiber, they fill you up, stabilize your blood sugars, and reduce cravings for bad foods. Balance your healthy weight loss plan by exercising a few days each week, avoiding late-night eating, and drinking plenty of water. After you lose the weight, you can switch gears into maintenance mode, having just one green smoothie per day as a replacement meal or snack. Stay active with regular exercise and keep making good food choices.

How Can I Gain Weight on Green Smoothies?

To gain weight by drinking green smoothies, increase the calorie content. Fats contain twice as many calories as protein or carbs. Choose fats that are cholesterol-free and high in nutrients.

Here are some healthy fats to add to your green smoothie:

- **1 cup pureed avocado:** 387 calories
- **4 tablespoons avocado oil:** 496 calories
- **4 tablespoons coconut oil:** 468 calories
- **4 tablespoons raw cashew butter:** 376 calories
- **4 tablespoons raw tahini (sesame paste):** 344 calories

Replace water with homemade almond milk as the liquid base of your smoothies to get another healthy hit of fat calories (Chapter 6 has instructions for making almond milk at home).

You can add a few extra dates to increase the calorie count of your smoothie, too. For example, one pitted Medjool date is 66 calories, so adding four Medjool dates to your green smoothie gives you an extra 264 calories. Combine dates with one of the added fats in this section, and you have a calorie-packed health drink to literally pump up the volume!

 Drink an extra green smoothie about an hour before bed to help you gain weight faster. Have one green smoothie before or after your workout for a power boost and/or recovery drink, and make an additional smoothie to drink before bed as a healthy calorie-loading snack.

How Do I Get More Protein, Iron, and Calcium in My Smoothies?

Luckily, green smoothies are already naturally high in protein, iron, and calcium. And the blended form of green smoothies makes it easier for your body to digest and absorb all the valuable nutrients.

You can boost the protein, iron, and calcium content even more by using naturally high sources of each in your smoothie:

 ✔ **Protein:** Focus on hemp seeds, chia seeds, ground flaxseed, sunflower seeds, almond butter, tahini, and/or spirulina powder.

 ✔ **Iron:** Add cherries, dried organic apricots, molasses, and more leafy greens (both powdered and whole-food forms).

 ✔ **Calcium:** Use homemade almond milk, beet greens, bok choy, collard greens, dandelion greens, kale, turnip greens, and spinach.

Why Do I Feel Gas and Bloating after My Green Smoothie?

If you've been eating a diet high in refined or processed foods or only heavy foods or cooked foods, drinking a blended smoothie full of raw fruits and greens can be a bit of a shock to the system. Technically speaking, your stomach may actually be low in digestive acids, or you may have an imbalance of gut bacteria. The result is excess gas and bloating as your stomach tries to correct itself and find a healthy balance.

If you feel bloated after your green smoothie, reduce the amount of leafy greens in each recipe by one-third. You can also add a probiotic capsule to your smoothie to bring in more good gut bacteria. As you start to feel better, slowly start adding more greens. Listen to your body and go at your own pace as you eventually increase the greens to the recipe amounts.

You can also try to reduce the amount of fruit you're using, and make sure you're not mixing too much fat and fruit. For example, if you're mixing avocado and Medjool dates and feeling really bloated, try removing the dates and see whether things improve. Finding what combinations work best for you may take some trial and error.

Do I Have to Use Greens in My Green Smoothie?

You can make a smoothie without greens, but then it's not a green smoothie! Remember, the whole point of having a green smoothie is to get more leafy greens into your diet. The benefit of drinking your greens is that it's easy to do every day, takes less than 5 minutes to prepare, and removes the guesswork about how to cook them. Most people eat some amount of fruit every day, but they're not eating enough greens. Enter the green smoothie as a viable solution that fits into your fast-paced modern-day busy life. You'll feel better; improve your hair, skin, and digestion; and increase your energy levels much faster if you add greens to your smoothies.

Can I Use Powdered Greens instead of Fresh Greens?

Nothing trumps a handful of fresh leafy greens in a green smoothie. Fresh is always best. But sometimes you just can't get fresh — such as when you're traveling or in winter months — and in that case, powdered greens are an excellent second choice.

If you really want to boost your nutrients, use both fresh greens and powdered greens year-round. I personally use spirulina or a green powder blend every day in addition to a variety of fresh greens. When traveling, I use only powdered greens. Be flexible to fit your health plan into real-world situations. Ultimately, a green smoothie with powdered greens is still better than no green smoothie at all!

Which Is Better: A Green Smoothie or a Green Juice?

Try not to think of in terms of which is "better" because green smoothies and green juices are both great for your health! Rather, consider which one is more practical for your busy lifestyle. You probably already have a blender at home, so your kitchen is already set up to start making green smoothies. Most people don't own a juicer and aren't that interested in buying another appliance.

In terms of the health benefits, both green smoothies and green juices offer a vast array of minerals, vitamins, and chlorophyll. The biggest difference between the two is that green smoothies still have all fiber intact, whereas juice has no fiber. A green smoothie can be made in advance and stored in the fridge for up to two days. Fresh juice needs to be consumed immediately. For more information on the difference between juice and smoothies, refer to Chapter 1.

Is It Possible to Drink Too Much Green Smoothie?

As long as you're integrating your green smoothies with a healthy diet, your body isn't going to let you drink "too much." Most of my students start drinking green smoothies and quickly feel that they're craving them. They often ask, "Can I drink more?" My answer is, "Of course!" When your body finally starts getting the nutrients it needs in a whole food form, you naturally feel like you want more. In the beginning, you may want one to two liters a day as your body gratefully accepts a new, easy-to-digest natural fuel. That's okay!

Green smoothies have a lot of natural fiber in them. Fiber in food fills you up and stops you from overeating. The refined flours and sugars in processed foods aren't filling, which is a reason why those foods are easy to overeat.

Over time, as you get all the nutrients you need, you may feel very satisfied with just one large glass of smoothie daily in addition to a healthy diet. Although you can do a green smoothie-only diet for a few days or even a few weeks as a great detox, you don't want to be on a liquid diet forever. A liquid-only diet isn't good for your teeth (they need to chew) and isn't sustainable for long-term health and well-being. Strive to have a healthy balance between drinking a smoothie every day and also chewing healthy food at other meals.

Do I Need to Take a Daily Vitamin if I'm Drinking Green Smoothies?

The short answer to this is that it depends. Drinking a green smoothie gives you a high boost of minerals and vitamins from real food with fiber, but you won't get everything from a green smoothie. For example, vitamin B12 occurs mostly in animal products and fortified (but processed) foods, so it won't be present in your smoothie. If your diet includes animal products, you may not need a B12 supplement, but for vegans and vegetarians, taking an additional B12 supplement is important. (Deficiency in vitamin B12 can cause fatigue, hair loss, and numbness in the fingers and toes.)

Here are some situations in which you may need a multivitamin in addition to having a green smoothie:

- ✔ While pregnant and/or breastfeeding
- ✔ After long travel to help your body recover more quickly
- ✔ During periods of high stress to minimize deficiency
- ✔ After illness or surgery to strengthen your immune system
- ✔ In winter months when you have less access to fresh food

Incorporating a variety of fruits and greens into your smoothie recipes helps cover your bases with the other nutrients your body needs. I personally don't take a multivitamin, but I make a point to use different fruits and different greens in my smoothies. I also switch between ground flaxseed and chia seeds for alternate sources of omega-3 fatty acids. And I use the same idea with variety in my other meals throughout the week, eating different veggies, nuts, seeds, grains, and healthy fats. If you follow this approach, you don't need to take a daily vitamin. Instead, spend your money on quality food.

Do Green Smoothies Work against Cellulite?

Green smoothies offer you a unique and powerful combination of chlorophyll, fiber, minerals, and added hydration that allows your skin to detoxify, repair, rebuild, and emit a youthful, healthy glow. The cause of cellulite is basically weak collagen, excess fat accumulation, and a buildup of toxins. As you age, collagen production declines and weakening of the skin occurs.

Dark leafy green vegetables contain powerful antioxidants that naturally help your skin produce more collagen. Fresh fruits are high in antioxidants and vitamin C, giving even more of a collagen-producing effect. Add to that some flaxseed or chia seeds for omega-3 fatty acids and fresh aloe vera to help repair and rejuvenate the skin, and you'll quickly start seeing results.

Appendix

Metric Conversion Guide

• •

Note: The recipes in this book weren't developed or tested using metric measurements. There may be some variation in quality when converting to metric units.

Common Abbreviations

Abbreviation(s)	What It Stands For
cm	Centimeter
C., c.	Cup
G, g	Gram
kg	Kilogram
L, l	Liter
lb.	Pound
mL, ml	Milliliter
oz.	Ounce
pt.	Pint
t., tsp.	Teaspoon
T., Tb., Tbsp.	Tablespoon

Volume

U.S. Units	Canadian Metric	Australian Metric
¼ teaspoon	1 milliliter	1 milliliter
½ teaspoon	2 milliliters	2 milliliters
1 teaspoon	5 milliliters	5 milliliters
1 tablespoon	15 milliliters	20 milliliters
¼ cup	50 milliliters	60 milliliters
⅓ cup	75 milliliters	80 milliliters
½ cup	125 milliliters	125 milliliters
⅔ cup	150 milliliters	170 milliliters
¾ cup	175 milliliters	190 milliliters
1 cup	250 milliliters	250 milliliters
1 quart	1 liter	1 liter
1½ quarts	1.5 liters	1.5 liters
2 quarts	2 liters	2 liters
2½ quarts	2.5 liters	2.5 liters
3 quarts	3 liters	3 liters
4 quarts (1 gallon)	4 liters	4 liters

Weight

U.S. Units	Canadian Metric	Australian Metric
1 ounce	30 grams	30 grams
2 ounces	55 grams	60 grams
3 ounces	85 grams	90 grams
4 ounces (¼ pound)	115 grams	125 grams
8 ounces (½ pound)	225 grams	225 grams
16 ounces (1 pound)	455 grams	500 grams (½ kilogram)

Length

Inches	Centimeters
0.5	1.5
1	2.5
2	5.0
3	7.5
4	10.0
5	12.5
6	15.0
7	17.5
8	20.5
9	23.0
10	25.5
11	28.0
12	30.5

Temperature (Degrees)

Fahrenheit	Celsius
32	0
212	100
250	120
275	140
300	150
325	160
350	180
375	190
400	200

(continued)

(continued)

Fahrenheit	Celsius
425	220
450	230
475	240
500	260

Index

About the Author

Jennifer Thompson is a fully trained and qualified Certified Comprehensive Iridologist (CCI) through the International Iridology Practitioner's Association (IIPA). She uses her background and education as a systems engineer to always look at the body as a whole in both understanding the true nature of imbalance and disease as well as making recommendations for improvement and healing.

After suffering from a full-body itchy rash that went undiagnosed by doctors for more than two years, Jennifer embarked on an elimination diet and subsequently determined the cause of her rash — a reaction to certain chemical additives in food. This discovery is what led her to a raw-food organic chemical-free diet.

For more than 16 years, Jennifer has been working with detox, raw foods, juice fasting, cleansing, and natural healing. In Koh Samui, Thailand, the world's largest detox destination, she worked with up to 150 people per day doing various fasting, colon cleansing, and juicing programs. She developed her green smoothie class for detox clients who were looking for fast and easy ways to cleanse and stay healthy back at home. Jennifer eventually traveled all over Asia teaching her green smoothie class to expats and health enthusiasts.

After leaving Asia in 2012, Jennifer moved her business online and built a substantial community of 50,000 followers on Twitter, offering daily nutrition tips and sharing success stories with raw food, detox, and natural healing. Her website http://healthybliss.net provides iridology analyses to clients and professional health coaching via Skype as well as detox and cleansing support. She also shares a wealth of information on raw food recipes, food additives, food allergies, emotional cleansing, and healthy living. Through Facebook, YouTube, Instagram, and Twitter, Jennifer educates, motivates, and inspires thousands of people all over the world on their journeys of healing.

Jennifer now works as a certified iridology practitioner, detox expert, health coach, and raw food educator. When she's not working with clients online, she travels the globe teaching and sharing her knowledge. She has worked with clients and presented workshops at various health and detox spas around the world, including The Four Seasons Maui, The Four Seasons in Koh Samui, Thailand, The Mandarin Oriental Hotel in Hong Kong, China, and Kamalaya Resort in Koh Samui, Thailand. She has also worked in Australia, Indonesia, Malaysia, Korea, Japan, Dubai, Jordan, Israel, Panama, Ecuador, and Costa Rica. Jennifer is currently based in the Middle East where she enjoys the warm Mediterranean climate and fantastic fresh fruits and local greens available for delicious green smoothies.

Connect with Jennifer online at http://healthybliss.net, www.facebook.com/rawfoodbliss, and https://twitter.com/rawfoodbliss.

Dedication

To my parents, who never wavered in their love and support as I went from Ivy League graduate to corporate engineer to round-the-world adventure traveler and finally to detox expert, raw food coach, health educator, and motivational speaker. I know it wasn't the path that you expected, but it's only because of you that I had the courage to blaze my own trail, walk where no one had gone, and leave a path for others to follow. Thank you, Mom and Dad, for letting me find my own way.

Author's Acknowledgments

Special appreciation to all of my green smoothie clients, students, friends, and followers from http://healthybliss.net. Your success stories inspire and motivate me to keep doing what I do. It's truly an honor and a pleasure to be part of your health journey!

Thanks to Tracy Boggier, my acquisitions editor, for inviting me to write this book and guiding me through the process across opposite sides of the globe. When Tracy first contacted me, I had just finished traveling the world for 1½ years and I thought all of the adventure was behind me. In reality, a whole new world of adventure began, and I am forever grateful that you believed in me to do the job. Sincerest thanks to my project editor, Elizabeth Rea, for taking on this project at a moment's notice and supporting me every step of the way. Your expertise and attention to detail is very much appreciated! And extra thanks to the copy editor, Megan Knoll, as well as the technical editor, recipe tester, and nutritional analyst for your behind-the-scenes roles in polishing my text and providing extremely valuable feedback.

A special thanks to my dearest friend Nancy, who helped to keep me sane through the process of writing this book by sending me daily emails to make me laugh and help me appreciate the smallest things in life. Although I didn't manage to get a recipe with your name in it, I can dedicate this small space to you. Heartfelt thanks to Yossi for not judging my strange fruit and vegetable diet, for jumping into my life with an open mind, and for actually turning into a great raw food vegan chef and a constant pillar of support. Thanks to my friends and family for your encouragement and for your understanding during all the times I had to say "no" and "I can't." I'm looking forward to getting away from the computer and going on some nature walks with all of you very soon!

Publisher's Acknowledgments

Acquisitions Editor: Tracy Boggier

Project Editor: Elizabeth Rea and Chad R. Sievers

Copy Editor: Megan Knoll

Technical Editor: Cathy M. Simpson

Recipe Tester: Emily Nolan

Nutritional Analysis: Angie Scheetz

Illustrator: Liz Kurtzman

Photographer: T.J. Hine

Stylist: Lisa Bishop

Art Coordinator: Alicia B. South

Project Coordinator: Lauren Buroker

Cover Photos: ©iStockphoto.com/ tashka2000